GW00708095

THE MAUDSLEY
Maudsley Monographs

MAUDSLEY MONOGRAPHS

HENRY MAUDSLEY, from whom the series of monographs takes its name, was the founder of The Maudsley Hospital and the most prominent English psychiatrist of his generation. The Maudsley Hospital was united with the Bethlem Royal Hospital in 1948 and its medical school, renamed the Institute of Psychiatry at the same time, became a constituent part of the British Postgraduate Medical Federation. It is now associated with King's College, London, and entrusted with the duty of advancing psychiatry by teaching and research. The Bethlem-Maudsley NHS Trust, together with the Institute of Psychiatry, are jointly known as The Maudsley.

The monograph series reports work carried out at The Maudsley. Some of the monographs are directly concerned with clinical problems; others, less obviously relevant, are in scientific fields that are cultivated for the furtherance of psychiatry.

Editor
Professor Sir David Goldberg MA DM MSc FRCP FRCPsych DPM
Assistant Editors
Professor A S David MPhil MSc FRCP MRCPsych MD
Dr T Wykes BSc PhD MPhil

Previous Editors	
1955-1962	Professor Sir Aubrey Lewis LLD DSc MD FRCP and Professor G W Harris MA MD DSc FRS
1962-1966	Professor Sir Aubrey Lewis LLD DSc MD FRCP
1966-1970	Professor Sir Denis Hill MB FRCP FRCPsych DPM and Professor J T Eayrs PhD DSc
1970-1979	Professor Sir Denis Hill MB FRCP FRCPsych DPM and Professor G S Brindley MD FRCP FRS
1979-1981	Professor G S Brindley MD FRCP FRS and Professor G F M Russell MD FRCP FRC(ED) FRCPsych
1981-1983	Professor G F M Russell MD FRCP FRCP(ED) FRCPsych
1983-1989	Professor G F M Russell MD FRCP FRCP(ED) FRCPsych and Professor E Marley MA MD DSc FRCP FRCPsych DPM
1989-1993	Professor G F M Russell MD FRCP FRCP(ED) FRCPsych and Professor B H Anderton BSc PhD

Maudsley Monographs number forty-one

Culture and Common Mental Disorders in Sub-Saharan Africa

Vikram Patel

*Clinical Research Fellow (Lecturer), Section of Epidemiology and General Practice, Institute of Psychiatry, DeCrespigny Park, London SE5 8AF, UK
(formerly Visiting Lecturer, Department of Psychiatry, University of Zimbabwe Medical School, Harare, Zimbabwe)*

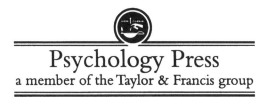

Psychology Press
a member of the Taylor & Francis group

Copyright © 1998 by Psychology Press Ltd
a member of the Taylor & Francis Group
All rights reserved. No part of this book may be reproduced in any form, by photostat, microform, retrieval system, or any other means without the prior written permission of the publisher.

Psychology Press Ltd, Publishers
27 Church Road
Hove
East Sussex, BN3 2FA
UK

British Library Cataloguing in Publication Data

A catalogue record for this book is available from the British Library

ISBN 0-86377-516-0
ISSN 0076-5465

Typeset by Quorum Technical Services Ltd, Cheltenham
Printed and bound in the UK by Biddles Ltd., Guildford and King's Lynn

To Bharati and Gauri

Contents

Glossary of abbreviations and Shona terms

ABBREVIATIONS

BDQ: Brief Disability Questionnaire
CISR: Revised Clinical Interview Schedule
CMD: Common mental disorders
CPN: Community psychiatric nurse
EMI: Explanatory model interview
FGD: Focus group discussions
GP: General practitioner
PHC: Primary health care clinics
SRQ: Self-reporting Questionnaire
SSQ: Shona Symptom Questionnaire
TMP: Traditional medical practitioner
VHW: Village health worker

FREQUENTLY USED SHONA TERMS

kufungisisa: Thinking too much
mamhepo: "Bad airs"
mudzimu: Ancestral spirits
muroyi: Witchcraft
n'anga: Traditional healer
profita: Faith healer

Acknowledgements

The work described in this monograph was supported by two principal grants. The Beit Medical Fellowships provided personal support and allowed me to stay in Zimbabwe for two years (August 1993–August 1995) conducting the field work and coordinating the project. The International Development Research Centre (Canada) provided a generous two year grant which supported all other project expenses and extended it well into 1996 and facilitated the completion of an outcome study and the dissemination of findings to health care providers and policy makers in Zimbabwe. Two other bodies provided small but important contributions: the German Technical Cooperation (GTZ, Harare) gave a grant to enable the field work to begin within months of my arriving in Harare; and Blair Research Laboratories (Zimbabwe Ministry of Health) funded two smaller projects, one of which helped to establish a sampling frame of TMP in the study areas.

I am indebted to my field research colleagues without whom none of the data collection would have been possible. In particular Fungisai Gwanzura and Essie Simunyu became indispensable colleagues and friends. Others who helped included Tecla Butau, Pat Maramba, and Tarisai Musara. The task of translation involved all these persons. In addition, Sekai Nhiwatiwa, Primrose Manyika, Edward Gushiri, Charles Singende, Jane Mutambirwa, and Gertrude Khumalo-Sakatukwa provided assistance. I am grateful to Dr O. Mbengeranwa, Director of the City of Harare Health Department and Professor G. Chavunduka,

Secretary-General of Zimbabwe National Traditional Healers Association for allowing us access to their respective health care facilities. Most of all, I am indebted to the nurses and TMPs who enthusiastically participated in every stage of the project and provided some of the insights which made my work in Zimbabwe a fascinating voyage of learning.

I am grateful to my colleagues in the University of Zimbabwe who provided support, advice, and encouragement. In particular, Mark Winston and Charles Todd were good friends and sources of constant intellectual stimulation. Professor Wilson Acuda provided supervision; Jane Mutambirwa and Alfred Chingono advised regarding the ethnographic components of the research; Professor Lincoln Moses, Simba Rusakaniko, and S. Siziya gave statistical advice; and Paul Linde, Laurie Schultz, Sunanda Ray, Farai Madzimbamuto, Bob Kitchin, Lawrence Hipshman, and Val Thorpe became sparring partners and friends. In London, Glyn Lewis, Martin Prince, Paulo Menezes, and Graham Dunn advised me on study design and statistics.

Most of all, I am grateful to two people. Anthony Mann provided unstinting support to my ideas, yet consistently smoothed my rough edges as my interest in a culturally sensitive epidemiology has evolved. Second, I owe an immeasurable amount of gratitude to my wife, Gauri, who has travelled with me while letting her own career drift. She has been my strongest critic and my closest friend through the years and, for us, the two years in Zimbabwe are already amongst the best times of our lives.

I wish to acknowledge the permission of the editors of journals in which some of the material in this monograph was published: *Psychological Medicine* (for the Ethnographic and Phenomenology Studies), *Acta Psychiatrica Scandinavica*, *Central African Journal of Medicine*, and *Social Psychiatry and Psychiatric Epidemiology* (material from the SSQ study) and the *British Journal of Psychiatry* (the Case-Control Study).

Abstract

Common Mental Disorders (CMD) are amongst the most frequent disorders in primary care attenders. They are characterised by the clinical presentation of somatic symptoms, anxiety, and depression and are associated with significant disability. In Africa, as in many other low-income regions, epidemiological research has almost entirely consisted of cross-sectional surveys of prevalence rates using methodologies and diagnostic models developed by European and American researchers. Traditional medical practitioners (TMP), who are amongst the key primary health care providers in Africa, have rarely been included in epidemiological studies. Despite these limitations, research has demonstrated a high prevalence of psychiatric morbidity in community and primary care settings. In contrast, ethnographic research has usually focused on descriptive studies with small numbers of TMPs. Such research has revealed a range of causal beliefs and types of mental illnesses in Africa. The principal limitation of the ethnographic approach has been the lack of a link with practical issues related to mental health services. The investigation of psychological disorders across cultures needs to blend both epidemiological and ethnographic approaches to ensure that research is not only sensitive to the local culture but is also relevant to mental health service development and is communicable across cultures.

This monograph begins by reviewing the key concepts and literature on cross-cultural psychiatric epidemiology, and the epidemiological and ethnographic literature on CMD in Sub-Saharan Africa. The overall objectives of the research studies described in the monograph were to obtain a complete picture of CMD in primary care attenders in Harare, Zimbabwe, using the existing literature and contemporary theory as a guide for developing its methodology. The research adopted a sequential design involving four distinct field research stages. Thus, this monograph departs from the trend of many before it in that it focuses not on one specific research study but on a series of four consecutive distinct studies linked with each other as the objectives evolved from ethnographic descriptions to epidemiological measurements. The aims of the Ethnographic Study were to describe the concepts of mental illness of a diverse range of primary health care providers and to elicit constructs of illness whose relationship to biomedical concepts of CMD could be examined. Next, in the Phenomenology Study, screening criteria elicited in the Ethnographic Study and the clinical assessment of primary health care providers were used to identify primary care attenders with conspicuous psychiatric morbidity. This study elicited the idioms of distress and explanatory models of these primary care attenders. The Shona Symptom Questionnaire Study involved the development and evaluation of the psychometric properties of a measure of CMD derived from the idioms of distress elicited in the previous study. This measure was then used as a case finding instrument in the final study, the Case–Control Study, which investigated the risk factors and associations of CMD. TMPs and primary health clinics were involved in all four studies while general practitioners were also involved in the Case–Control Study, reflecting the pluralistic nature of primary health care in Africa.

The outcome of these studies includes a description of the concepts of mental illness held by a diverse group of health care providers and the description of the explanatory models of illness experience of persons with conspicuous psychiatric morbidity. The Shona Symptom Questionnaire, a 14-item questionnaire for the detection and measurement of CMD in the Shona language, was developed and its reliability and validity demonstrated. The studies demonstrated that the prevalence of CMD was greater amongst attenders at TMP as compared to PHC and that two indigenous models of illness (thinking too much or *kufungisisa* and the model of supernatural causation) were closely related to the biomedical construct of CMD. The relationship between different criteria for determining the presence of a psychological disorder, for example those based on biomedical models and those based on local care provider concepts, were examined. The Case–Control Study demonstrated that female gender, economic impoverishment, infertility, and disability were strongly associated with CMD; this study replicated the association between the two indigenous constructs of illness and CMD. In the discussion, material from all four studies is brought together to explore the contribution of culture to the presentation, assessment, classification, and risk factors for CMD in primary care in Harare. In the final analysis, this book attempts to present an innovative and pragmatic approach to the investigation of psychological disorders across cultures.

The relationship of culture, political structures, and ethnicity are a confusing and complex area. When one refers to the dominant paradigms in psychiatry, it is obvious that the major influences have originated from Europe and the USA. In attempting to use a phrase which denotes this dominant influence, I have had to consider a range of words: "Western nations" was considered inappropriate due to the complex ethnic mixture of these societies; and "industrialised societies" was dropped due to the rapid industrialisation affecting many hitherto less developed societies. Two terms are used in the book when referring to two concepts with some overlap: "biomedical" is used when referring to the medical model of psychiatry, such as current international classifications. However, it is recognised that this term does not exclude the fact that the movement for a more culturally sensitive epidemiology has substantial biomedical roots. "Euro-American cultures" is used when referring to European and American systems of thought about mental illness which form the dominant paradigm behind current biomedical classifications. The limitations of this term are recognised in that much of cross-cultural psychiatry has been driven by researchers from Euro-American cultures.

CHAPTER ONE

Introduction

THE "NEW" CROSS-CULTURAL PSYCHIATRY

Epidemiology is of particular importance in psychiatry for several reasons: first, mental health resources are insufficient and epidemiological research can help establish the scale of the need by describing the frequency of psychiatric disorders and the burden they pose on individuals, families, and health care systems; second, most psychiatric disorders are poorly understood and epidemiological research can help unravel the multi-factorial aetiology of these disorders; third, epidemiological research can help improve our understanding of the relationship between physical and psychological illness (Tansella, de Girolamo, & Sartorius, 1992).

Historically, cross-cultural studies in psychiatric epidemiology have suffered several problems. First, case identification techniques varied from site to site and methods were not standardised (Compton et al., 1991). These inconsistencies led to a movement to standardise the process of psychiatric measurement and diagnosis. This process of standardisation was driven by psychiatric classification systems originating in Euro-American societies. Standardised interviews which mimicked the clinical psychiatric evaluation were developed and became the criteria for determining "caseness" in epidemiological investigations (Williams, Tarnopolsky, & Hand, 1980). After standardisation in Euro-American cultures, the interviews were subsequently used in other cultures. Most of these subsequent cross-cultural psychiatric investigations relied on implicit, largely untested assumptions: (1) the universality of mental illnesses, implying that regardless of cultural variations, disorders as described in Euro-American classifications occur everywhere; (2) invariance, implying that the core features of psychiatric syndromes are invariant; and (3) validity, implying that although refinement is possible, the diagnostic categories of current classifications are valid clinical constructs (Beiser, Cargo, & Woodbury, 1994). This approach, termed as the "etic" or universalist approach, became the most popular method for epidemiological investigations of mental illness across cultures. The etic approach offered the perspective that, since mental illness was similar throughout the world, psychiatric taxonomies, their measuring instruments, and models of health care were also globally applicable. There are two dominant systems of psychiatric classification, the ICD-10 Classification of Mental and Behavioural Disorders (World Health Organisation, 1992) and the Diagnostic and Statistical Manual (American Psychiatric Association, 1985), which reflect the psychiatric nosologies of Euro-American medicine. Diagnostic criteria of syndromes can and do change over time as is well demonstrated by the regular revisions of international psychiatric classifications; these revisions are considerably influenced by attitudinal, political, and historical factors (Westermeyer, 1985). Some cross-cultural researchers and psychiatric researchers in low-income countries have argued for the effectiveness and universal applicability of current classification systems (e.g. Corin & Murphy, 1979; Kerson & Jones, 1988; Odejide, 1979; Sen & Mari, 1987).

Problems with the etic approach arose when cross-cultural researchers pointed out that there was risk of confounding culturally distinctive behaviour with psychopathology on the basis of superficial similarities of behaviour patterns or phenomena in different cultures (Draguns, 1984). It was argued that classification of psychiatric disorders largely reflected American and European concepts of psychopathology based on implicit cultural concepts of normality and deviance (Baskin, 1984; Kirmayer, 1989). Some argued that cross-cultural psychiatry should examine the influence of culture on mental illness in Euro-American society itself, rather than assume that these illnesses were "natural" and free of any cultural bias (Murphy, 1977). Critics accused the etic approach of contributing to a world view which "privileges biology over culture" (Eisenbruch, 1991) and ignoring the cultural and social contexts of psychiatric disorders.

The field of medical anthropology has exerted a growing influence on health research, particularly in low-income countries. This influence has seen a shift in paradigms in public health and epidemiology from its unifocal and positivist "scientific" approach to the recognition that illness is the result of a "web of causation" which includes the individual's sociocultural environment (Heggenhougen & Draper, 1990). Medical anthropology has been one of the key factors which fuelled the development of the "emic" approach in cross-cultural psychiatry. At a general level this approach argued that the culture-bound aspects of biomedicine, such as its emphasis on medical disease entities, limited its universal applicability (Helman, 1991). More specifically, this approach argued that culture played such an influential role in the presentation of psychiatric disorders that it was wrong to presume a priori that Euro-American psychiatric categories were appropriate throughout the world (Littlewood, 1990). Part of this argument was based on the lack of specific pathophysiological changes which could be identified in psychiatric disorders, which effectively made the diagnostic categories "illnesses" as compared to "diseases" (Helman, 1981; Littlewood, 1991). The emic approach proposed to evaluate phenomena from within a culture and its context, aiming to understand its significance and relationship with other intracultural elements.

Purely emic studies have also drawn their share of criticism, the most fundamental one being that they are unable to provide data which can be compared across cultures (Mari, Sen, & Cheng, 1989). These studies are usually small in scale and are unable to resolve questions of the long-term course and treatment outcome of illness episodes (Kirmayer, 1989). The reliability of emic studies is in doubt due to the lack of standardisation of research methods and the biased findings based on the interpretations of individual researchers. The emic approach has been criticised for not suggesting plausible alternatives, such as a set of principles which would help ensure cultural sensitivity, or models upon which to fashion culturally sensitive nosologies (Beiser et al., 1994). It is argued that culture is not a static concept; all cultures are constantly evolving and changing and with the increasing influence of Euro-American values and urbanisation in many low-income societies, "traditional" beliefs may not be as rigidly held as is supposed. Furthermore, any individual may hold a multiplicity of ideas regarding his illness and any or all of these ideas may change with time (Eisenbruch, 1990).

Despite major strides in the international classification of mental disorders and in the ethnographic approach to studying mental illness, a truly international psychiatry does not exist (Westermeyer, 1989). Thus, there are strengths and weaknesses of both the etic and emic approaches in cross-cultural psychiatry. It is increasingly accepted that the integration of their methodological strengths is essential for the development of the "new cross-cultural psychiatry" or a culturally sensitive psychiatry (Kleinman, 1987; Littlewood, 1990). Value must be given to both folk beliefs about mental illness as well as to the biomedical system of psychiatry (Leff, 1990). It is important to investigate the patients' "explanatory models", i.e. how patients understand their problems, their nature, origin, consequences, and remedies since these can radically assist patient–doctor negotiations over appropriate treatment (Kleinman, 1980). Similarly, researchers should examine the psychiatric symptoms of persons who are considered to be mentally ill by the local population and to interview the TMPs and other primary carers to ascertain the diagnostic systems used. In essence, the central aim of the "new" cross-cultural psychiatry would be to describe mental illness in different cultures using methods which are sensitive and valid for the local culture and resulting in data which are comparable across cultures. In order to tackle this difficult task, psychiatric research needs to blend both ethnographic and epidemiological methods and emphasise the unique contribution of both approaches to the understanding of mental illness across cultures.

COMMON MENTAL DISORDERS (CMD)

This is a term coined by Goldberg and Huxley (1992) to describe "disorders which are commonly encountered in community settings, and whose occurrence signals a breakdown in normal functioning." CMD, also referred to as non-psychotic mental disorders, encompass a broad group of distress states which manifest with a mixture of anxiety and depressive symptoms. CMD are the contemporary equivalent of the neuroses, a descriptive category which has become increasingly unpopular because of its vague meaning and stigma. CMD have been classified in ICD-10 in two main categories: "neurotic, stress-related and somatoform disorders" with a number of subcategories and "mood disorders" (with specific reference to unipolar depression). A simpler classification of CMD has been devised for use in primary health care (Ustun et al., 1995b; see Table 1.1).

In practice, the subcategories of CMD are not without their conceptual problems: for example, obsessive–compulsive disorders are not common in community settings, whereas phobic disorders may not be counted as

TABLE 1.1
Classification of common mental disorders for primary health care in ICD-10

F32	Depression
F40	Phobic disorder
F41.0	Panic disorder
F41.1	Generalised anxiety
F41.2	Mixed anxiety and depression
F43	Adjustment disorder
F44	Dissociative disorder
F45	Unexplained somatic symptoms
F48	Neurasthenia
F51	Sleep problems

mental illnesses by some investigators. Part of this problem may be accounted for by the fact that classifications have tended to reflect the results of psychiatric assessments at tertiary care level. In most primary care patients, symptoms of anxiety and depression coexist to such an extent that their categorisation in either group is difficult. The WHO multinational study of CMD found that for all specific psychiatric disorders (excluding alcohol dependence), comorbidity rates (with other psychiatric disorders) exceeded 50% (Ormel et al., 1994) suggesting that one of the basic criteria of a successful classification, i.e. the mutual exclusiveness of different categories, was not achieved. Indeed, Goldberg and Huxley (1992) state that "it is becoming clear that the idea that CMD should be thought of as discrete disease entities with distinct causes, course and treatment is probably untenable."

The World Health Report based on 1993 statistics shows that neurotic, stress-related and somatoform disorders are the third most frequent causes of morbidity (prevalence rates) worldwide (WHO, 1995). CMD are an important cause of disability and have been identified as a significant public health problem (Blue & Harpham, 1994; World Bank, 1993). The multinational study of the prevalence, nature and determinants of CMD was conducted in 14 countries, including Nigeria in Africa (Ustun & Sartorius, 1995). The startling finding of this study was that, despite the use of standardised methods in all centres, there were enormous variations in most variables. Indeed, the only similarities across centres were the general observations of the ubiquity of CMD and the comorbidity of anxiety and depression and the association of CMD and disability even after adjustment for physical disease severity. On the other hand, specific variables showed substantial variations; thus the prevalence rates of CMD ranged from 7% to 52% of primary care attenders; physician recognition of CMD varied from 5% to nearly 60%; and the association of key variables such as gender, physical ill health, and education with CMD were opposite in different centres (Goldberg & Lecrubier, 1995). For example, the relative risk of having a CMD for females varied from 1.9 in Bangalore to 0.3 in Ibadan. Similarly, the relative risk for depressive disorder for those with two or more children varied from 3.3 in Athens to 0.19 in Ibadan. These marked variations suggest the need for regional studies with local health service-driven priorities to complement multinational studies with their emphasis on uniformity and universality (Patel & Winston, 1994).

CULTURE AND COMMON MENTAL DISORDERS

Study of the influence of culture on mental illness is important for several reasons: for example, it enables us to understand how patients from different ethnic groups experience and express mental distress and, further, by shedding light on aetiological factors it plays an important role in the development of psychiatric theory by illuminating the diverse influences on mental distress posed by culture, society, and biology (Beiser, 1985; Sartorius, 1986). In recent years there has been increasing concern regarding the validity of cross-cultural psychiatric studies which have mainly utilised the etic approach. The uncertainty arises from the diagnosis of mental illness which relies almost entirely on clinical presentations, there being no "gold standard" validating pathological or diagnostic tests. It is generally accepted that culture plays a profound role in the expression of idioms of distress and that in psychiatry language is the very means of conveying symptoms. Yet, the validity of the descriptive categories of current classifications for other cultures has rarely been evaluated. The description of illnesses in Euro-American classifications are automatically assumed to be cross-culturally valid, prompting accusations of "psychiatric imperialism" (Fernando, 1991). Concerns about validity should be greatest for syndromes of depression and anxiety, where the boundaries between "normal sadness" and "clinical depression" are blurred (Kirmayer, 1989). For example, while the experience of normal sadness may be similar across cultures, the clinical significance of depression as a unique illness category may vary considerably (Beiser, 1985). On the other hand, it has been argued that dysphoria is a univeral human experience and that depression can be recognised in many cultures. Although there may be indigenous categories of mental illness, this does not necessarily invalidate the application of international psychiatric categories for epidemiological purposes (Bebbington, 1993).

The first problem one encounters in examining the cross-cultural validity of the clinical category of depression is that many languages have no conceptually equivalent term for depression (Chaturvedi, 1993; Ihezue, 1989; Manson, Shore, & Bloom, 1985; Swartz, Ben-Arie, & Teggin, 1985). Conceptualisation of depression in cross-cultural research is made especially difficult by the widely varying idioms of distress expressed by patients and the varying contextual significance of such idioms (Angst, 1973; Lutz, 1985). It cannot be assumed that even "core" features of depression in one culture have the same meaning in another. For example, Obeyesekere (1985) argues that hopelessness, a core cognitive feature of the biomedical model of depression, is perceived to be a positive feature of mental state for Buddhists. Although some African studies have reported that the "core" symptoms of depression were the same in their patients, these researchers sampled patients who were attending psychiatric facilities or who had already been diagnosed as having a depressive disorder by psychiatrists (Keegstra, 1986; Majodina & Attah Johnson, 1983; Makanjuola & Olaifa, 1987); it is unclear whether these patients were representative of depression in the community.

Somatic symptoms have often been percieved to be a common mode of presentation of depression in low-income countries. Recent studies have shown that, contrary to popular belief, somatic presentations of depression were also common in Euro-American societies (Bridges & Goldberg, 1985). Thus, somatic symptoms of depression appeared to be universal to many cultures, though this did not imply that the appropriate name for the disorder was "depression", but merely that in Euro-American cultures the everyday experience of sadness came to the fore to the point that it became the most characteristic feature of "depression". It has been suggested that somatisation is "an expression of personal and social distress in an idiom of bodily complaints and medical help seeking" nonspecific to particular diagnoses (Kleinman & Kleinman, 1985). For example, Cheng's study in Taiwan (1989) suggests that for a substantial number of psychiatric patients in primary care, somatisation was a form of illness behaviour manifested in neurotic patients from a wide diagnostic spectrum including anxiety and depression.

Can depression be diagnosed in patients who do not experience the cognitive features of the illness? While some authors have assumed that depression is the "true" illness in patients presenting with nonspecific somatic symptoms (Ndetei & Muhangi, 1979), others have expressed reservations in diagnosing depression when the central cognitive features of the illness are absent (Venkoba Rao, 1994). Illness patterns with their own characteristic clinical and epidemiological features, but with no Euro-American equivalent, are seen to be "masked" presentations of an "underlying" depression. In these situations the fact that some patients complained of low mood or achieved "cut-off" scores on depression rating scales was taken as evidence for the assumption that the "true" diagnosis was depression, even though it is well recognised that emotional responses such as low mood and apprehension commonly occur as a reaction to a number of medical and psychiatric conditions. Thus, patients presenting with a primary complaint of "loss of semen" may also be depressed (Cheng, 1989); is depression comorbid with the semen loss syndrome (*dhat* syndrome in India), or is the latter a "masked" or "somatised" form of depression? Angst (1973) argues that the current concept of depression is so rooted in European culture that it is strongly influenced by a cultural bias; in his view, then, the concept of "masked depression" is as representative of a depressive syndrome as the classic descriptions.

Questions regarding the cross-cultural validity of the clinical category of depression remain unresolved, not least because "the universality of the category of depression (and other categories of neurotic disorder) is *assumed*, eliminating the need to establish validity, and the tautological circle is completed when the symptoms that serve as criteria for the diagnosis, because they are believed to reflect specific psychophysiological and hormonal states, are assumed to be universal" (Good, Good, & Moradi, 1985). Theoretic assumptions underlying the etic and emic approaches have influenced the choices researchers make of the method of assessment of psychiatric disorders across cultures. These methods will now be described.

ASSESSMENT OF MENTAL DISORDERS ACROSS CULTURES

The quantitative assessment of mental disorders, such as the measurement of psychiatric morbidity and determination of prevalence rates, requires standardised questionnaires. There are two methods of using question-naires across cultures, viz., using preexisting measures developed in other cultures or developing measures *de novo*. Most cross-cultural studies use instruments developed in one culture (to date, always a Euro-American culture), translate them, and apply them to another culture. Given the central importance of language in expressing symptoms, the translation of the instrument is perhaps the single most important step in etic studies. The translated version should be evaluated on a number of different parameters such as its content, technical, conceptual, and criterion equivalence (Flaherty et al., 1988; Krause, 1990; Sartorius, 1993). Apart from an emphasis on translation, it is important to evaluate the validity of instruments when they are to be used as case finding instruments. For example, though the Self-reporting Questionnaire (SRQ) is used by many authors with a standard cut-off score of 6–7, investigators who have evaluated its validity in Africa have shown that higher cut-off scores are more sensitive and specific for case identification (Kortmann & Ten-Horn, 1988; Patel & Todd, 1996). Although most studies using etic instruments deal superficially with the issue of translation and validity, there is a growing literature on research using etic instruments suitably translated and validated for use in different cultural settings. This research has shown that if careful attention is placed on the issues of validity and translation, etic instruments can be used with confidence across cultures (e.g. Bravo, Canino, Rubio-Stipec, & Woodbury-Farina, 1991; Manson et al., 1985; Mumford et al., 1991b).

There have been a few successful attempts at developing new methods of assessment for CMD which integrate emic and etic approaches both in Africa and elsewhere. The following are four examples of such studies from non-African settings. Kinzie et al. (1982) described the development of a Vietnamese language rating scale for depression. Items were derived from the Beck Depression Inventory, Vietnamese terms elicited from a lexicon generated by bilingual mental health workers, somatic symptoms frequently presented by Vietnamese patients, and items designed to tap the behavioural and somatic symptoms of depression. Of the 15 items which discriminated for depression 10 were unrelated to either lowered mood or the Western concept of depression. The Bradford Somatic Inventory (BSI) developed in the UK for use with patients from the Indian subcontinent (Mumford et al., 1991a) emphasised the important role of somatic symptoms in the expression of emotional distress. The BSI consisted of somatic symptoms recorded in the case notes of patients in the UK and Pakistan. These items were checked against the case notes of patients in India and Nepal and over 90% coverage of all somatic symptoms was achieved. The Urdu and English versions were then administered to bilingual students in Pakistan to determine linguistic equivalence. Conceptual equivalence was determined by studying the factor analysis of responses by patients with functional disorders in Britain and Pakistan. The seven-item Primary Care Psychiatric Questionnaire (PPQ) was developed in India (Srinivasan & Suresh, 1990; Suresh, Suresh Kumar, Bashyam, & Srinivasan, 1993) on the rationale that patients preferred to express their distress in somatic terms and primary health care staff were more comfortable in discussing such symptoms. Therefore, a screening measure consisting of somatic symptoms would be more appropriate for the Indian setting. Eleven symptoms frequently presented by patients with neurotic disorders were administered to a random sample of new primary care attenders. Seven symptoms which occurred more often in cases (as judged by a psychiatric interview) formed the PPQ. The Chinese Health Questionnaire (CHQ) was developed with the 30-item General Health Questionnaire as its starting point (Cheng & Williams, 1986; Goldberg, 1978). An additional 30 items based on the Chinese concepts of illness, such as the concern about the heat and coldness of food, were added. The resulting 60-item questionnaire was validated against a standardised psychiatric interview. The final questionnaire consisted of 12 items which discriminated cases best; half originated from the GHQ and the remainder were emic items.

In Africa, there are three published examples of attempts to develop culturally sensitive psychiatric instruments, all from West Africa. Beiser and colleagues' (1972, 1976) studies with the Serer people of Senegal began with ethnographic work setting the stage for eliciting a local taxonomy of mental illness and lexicon of Serer illness terms. A group of patients with "illnesses of the spirit" were interviewed showing that these illnesses were closely related to psychiatric concepts of mental illness. The research group further developed an interview schedule based on a preexisting questionnaire and the lexicon of illness terms. The Somatic Screening Instrument designed by Ebigbo (1982) in Nigeria was developed by listing complaints of patients diagnosed as suffering from anxiety neurosis. This questionnaire was then tested on a patient and control group to identify items with discriminant validity. Of the original 65 complaints, 46 were found to distinguish male cases from normals while 30 items distinguished female cases from normals. The Nigerian version of the SRQ was developed because many of the symptoms represented in the item content were found not to be presented spontaneously and were subject to considerable "yea-saying" bias. Ten "culture-specific" items were added to the SRQ and the 30-item version used with samples of cases of CMD and their relatives. The 20 items which discriminated best between these two groups went on to form the Nigerian SRQ-20 which contained nine "culture-specific" items (Martyns-Yellowe, 1995).

All the above methods were innovative in developing assessment measures by creating lists of items derived either entirely from idioms of distress or by adding these idioms to a preexisting questionnaire and then evaluating its validity using psychiatric diagnosis as elicited by clinical or standardised interview as the criterion.

EPIDEMIOLOGY OF MENTAL ILLNESS IN SUB-SAHARAN AFRICA

Perhaps the earliest attempt at a psychiatric epidemiology in Africa was the work of Carothers (1953) who reported that depression virtually never occurred in Africa and that this disorder was 13 times as common in the UK. His work was largely discredited since it was based on hospital populations and had racist overtones in his implication that the lack of depression was evidence of the underdevelopment of the African brain. Similar racist ideologies were evident from some researchers in South Africa; for example, Le Roux (1973) argued that the apparent lack of specific terms equivalent to European psychopathology suggested an "obvious ignorance" of the nature of such derangements and that this "primitiveness of the subconscious" could emerge as "physical assault". Studies in the late 1960s to the mid-1970s which used operationalised definitions of psychiatric disorder, structured questionnaires, and community or primary care samples of patients showed that psychiatric disorders were at least as common in Africa as in Euro-American societies (Binitie, 1981; Giel & Van Luijk, 1969; Gillis, Lewis, & Slabbert, 1968; Leighton et al., 1963).

Pyschiatric epidemiology in Africa has been reviewed by several authors in the recent past (German, 1987; Odejide, Oyewumi, & Ohaeri, 1989; Parry, 1996; Reeler, 1986). The objective of the review in this monograph is to provide a brief overview of research in primary care and community settings with a specific aim of evaluating the cultural sensitivity of the study methodology. Of the studies published since the mid-1970s, 14 were identified through bibliographic searches representing 8 Sub-Saharan African countries. Sub-Saharan Africa was selected as the geographical region for review (for both this and the following section) because its nations share numerous cultural and historical features distinct from those of predominantly Arab North Africa (Stock, 1995). A review of the study settings, methods, and key findings is presented in Table 1.2.

The prevalence of mental disorder was reported to be greater in both rural community studies as compared to similar studies in European or American settings. The rural Ugandan study in which researchers used methods identical to those used in a study in London reported that hypomanic disorders were more than five times as frequent, depressive disorders twice as frequent, and anxiety states three to four times as frequent amongst female respondents. In rural Lesotho, depression was four times as common and panic disorder was five times as common in both sexes when compared to data from the USA. On average, in both studies, more than one in four rural inhabitants were diagnosed as suffering from a current mental illness. Before accepting these findings, one must consider their validity and meaning to the community. To do so, one would need to elicit the patients' and care providers' views about the nature of the illness. Only the Ugandan study explicitly asked the patients' views about whether they thought they had a mental illness or any illness in the past involving the symptoms discussed during interview with the Present State Examination (PSE; Wing, Cooper, & Sartorius, 1974). The authors remarked that "it was fairly rare to get a positive answer, and negative answers were considered unreliable" (Orley & Wing, 1979). The relationship of psychiatric disorder and explanatory models in the Lesotho study was only presented for patients with a panic disorder. More than two-thirds of patients (68%) said they did not know the cause of their problem; 23% attributed psychological causes and only 3% mentioned spiritual causes. No explanation was provided for what a "psychological" cause or "spiritual" cause meant. Nearly three-quarters of patients (72%) did not know what the treatment would be and, perhaps surprisingly, not one patient said that a TMP might be helpful. This finding was at odds with the finding that nearly a quarter (23%) had sought traditional medical help for panic symptoms, casting some doubt on the reliability of the findings.

Prevalence rates in the PHC studies ranged from 10% to 69% with a median prevalence of 22.5% and a mean prevalence (excluding the one extreme prevalence figure of 69%) of 21.8%. In Zimbabwe, widely varying findings were reported ranging from an annual prevalence rate of mental disorder of 26% over a four-year study period (Hall & Williams, 1987) to a prevalence of 10% over a one-month study period (Reeler, Williams, &

TABLE 1.2

Epidemiological studies of mental disorder in primary care and community settings in Sub-Saharan Africa after 1978

Authors/Country	Setting	Sample size	Emic element/ translation	Stages	Interviews	Findings
1. Ndetei & Muhangi, 1979; Kenya	U PHC	140	No information	1	Clinical examination	Overall: 20% M 19%; F 22%
2. Orley & Wing, 1979; Uganda	R COM	221	Translation/back translation	1	PSE	Overall: 25% DEP: M 14.3%, F 22.6%, ANX: M 3.1%, F 4.3%
3. Harding et al., 1980; Sudan	R PHC	360	Brief data on translation	2	SRQ, PSE	Overall: 10.6%
4. Diop et al., 1982; Senegal	R PHC	933	No information	1	SRQ	Overall: 16.2%
5. Dhadphale et al., 1983; Kenya	SU/R OPD	388	Modified SPI item on bewitchment	2	SRQ, SPI	Overall 29% DEP 9.3%, ANX 8.5%, MDI 4.9%, SCZ 1.5%
6. Oduowle & Ogunyemi, 1984, Nigeria	U OPD	80	Translation/back translation	1	GHQ-30	Overall: 69%
7. de Jong et al., 1986; Guinea-Bissau	R PHC	251	Portuguese version of SRQ from Brazil	2	SRQ, PSE	Overall 12%
8. Hall & Williams, 1987; Zimbabwe	R OPD	448	No information	2	SRQ, PSE	Overall > 10% M=F
9. Dhadphale et al., 1989; Kenya	R OPD	881	No information	2	SRQ, SPI, HDRS	Overall 25% DEP 9%
10. Abiodun, 1989; Nigeria	R PHC	214	No information	1	PSE	Overall: 22.5% DEP 14%,
11. Hollifield et al., 1990; Lesotho	R/U COM	356	Translation/back translation	2	Short DIS, SCL-90	Overall: 22.8% DEP 12.4%; PD 11%,
12. Jegede et al., 1990, Nigeria	U OPD	104	Translation/back translation	1	PSE, Clinical interview, CES-D	Overall (PSE) 39.7% Overall (CES-D) 42% Overall (Clinical) 47.7%
13. Gureje & Obikoya, 1992, Nigeria	U PHC	787	Translation/back translation	2	Clinical interview, CES-D GHQ-12 and CIDI	Overall: 35.1% DEP 8.8%, GAD 9.1% Somatoform dis 16.7%
14. Reeler et al., 1993; Zimbabwe	R/U PHC/ OPD	1236	No information	1	SRQ	Overall: 26%

Key: R = rural; SU = semi-urban; U = urban; COM = community; OPD = hospital outpatient department; PHC = primary health clinic; DIS = - Diagnostic Interview Schedule; HDRS = Hamilton Depression Rating Scale; PSE = Present State Examination; SCL-90 = Symptom CheckList; SPI = Standard Psychiatric Interview; SRQ = Self Rating Questionnaire; GHQ-30 = 30-item General Health Questionnaire; CES-D = Centre for Epidemiological Studies of Depression Scale; CIDI = Composite International Diagnostic Interview; ANX = anxiety; DEP = depression; DYS = dysthymia; GAD = generalised anxiety disorder; MDI = manic depressive illness; PD = panic disorder; SCZ = schizophrenia.

Todd, 1993). Diagnostic breakdown was given in half the studies and showed that neurotic disorders were the commonest conditions in primary care and, of these, depression and anxiety were the commonest diagnoses. Phobic disorders, obsessive–compulsive disorders, and disassociative disorders were rarely, if ever, identified.

The most common presenting complaints in PHC attenders were somatic symptoms such as fever, headache, epigastric discomfort, abdominal and chest pains, cough, genito-urinary symptoms, and constipation; patients very rarely complained of "psychological symptoms". The authors of one study diagnosed depression and anxiety in patients who displayed none of the subjective cognitive symptoms of either (Ndetei & Muhangi, 1979). These authors suggested that in African culture "concepts like sadness and anxiety do not carry medical implications and so on a cultural level alone it is unlikely that patients would complain of these states." Three studies attempted to investigate the coexistence of common medical diseases or nutritional problems which are important causes of somatic morbidity in Sub-Saharan Africa (Gureje & Obikoya, 1992) but only one reported on comorbidity of physical illness, showing that a fifth of patients with a psychiatric disorder also suffered a physical illness (Abiodun, 1989).

Case recognition by health clinic staff was reported in five studies and was always found to be low. For example, in a Nigerian study, only 14.6% of morbidity was recognised by care providers (Abiodun, 1989), while in a Zimbabwean study, the figure was even lower at 4.2% (Hall & Williams, 1987). Patients with psychotic and suicidal symptoms were most likely to be recognised as having a mental illness, whereas those with somatic "equivalents" were least likely. All the studies which elicited the diagnostic assessment of the health care provider were doing so to examine how many "cases" were detected by them, rather than to determine their views as clinicians with much experience in primary care. Even though psychiatry in Africa is principally concerned with the "psychiatry of psychoses" (Asuni, 1991), the hospital-based psychiatric instruments designed in a foreign culture were the gold standards for diagnosis in community and primary care settings. Thus, even when neither the patient nor health clinic staff considered a mental illness to be present both were considered to be of secondary importance to, and less "reliable" than, the instrument.

Baasher (1982) noted the unique difficulties in conducting epidemiological investigations in low-income countries, such as organisational deficiencies, shortage of trained personnel and lack of reliable medical recording. Despite these problems, researchers in a number of African countries have successfully conducted epidemiological investigations and demonstrated that psychiatric morbidity is common in community and primary care populations. Some studies have also demonstrated that such disorders are often not recognised by primary care staff and others have noted that this may lead to inappropriate medication, unnecessary investigations, chronicity of morbidity, and dissatisfaction with health care services (Freeman, 1991). However, from the perspective of a culturally sensitive epidemiology, none of the 14 studies reviewed employed a significant emic element. All the intruments used were etic; the majority were developed in Britain. Only one study provided detailed information on translation and this study identified many linguistic and conceptual problems with the instrument used (PSE). Validity was rarely evaluated for the instruments. The SRQ was the most frequently used instrument. In the WHO study, which led to its development and described its use in four low-income nations, the cut-off score varied from 3–4 in one centre to 10–11 in another (Harding et al., 1980). Yet, all the African studies used a standard cut-off score of 6–7. Recent research has shown that higher cut-off scores, such as 9–10, are more appropriate for the SRQ in African settings (Kortmann & Ten Horn, 1988; Patel & Todd, 1996). Kortmann and Ten-Horn (1988) examined the validity of the SRQ in Ethiopia and found that the instrument lacked criterion validity, that many items lacked concept validity and that scores often reflected help-seeking behaviour rather than mental illness. Similarly, Martyns-Yellowe (1995) found that, in Nigeria, many of the SRQ items were not presented spontaneously and were subject to a yea-saying bias. Although the PSE was designed for use in hospital-based populations, the instrument was used in a number of studies without any mention of issues pertaining to its validity in community or primary care settings (Parry, 1996).

In conclusion, epidemiological studies in Africa have used the etic approach and none can be said to apply the principles of the new cross-cultural psychiatry. Despite the frequent observation that patients with CMD tend to consult TMP (Olatawura, 1982), none of the studies included TMP attenders. Forty years of psychiatric epidemiology in Africa have almost entirely focused on cross-sectional estimates of prevalence using imported methodologies with little attention to indigenous categories of mental illness, local symptom profiles, care provider diagnostic concepts and patient explanatory models.

EXPLANATORY MODELS OF MENTAL ILLNESS IN SUB-SAHARAN AFRICA

Explanatory models (EMs) is a term coined by Kleinman (1980) to denote the "notions about an episode of sickness and its treatment that are employed by all those engaged in the clinical process." EMs are formed from a variable cluster of cultural symbols, experiences and expectations associated with a particular category of illness. EMs reveal sickness labelling and cultural idioms for expressing the experiences of illness. Explanatory models of illness influence health seeking behaviour and health service utilization (Fosu, 1981). A review by the author covered work from 11 Sub-Saharan nations, viz., Nigeria, Senegal, Uganda, Zimbabwe, Botswana, Ethiopia, Ghana, Swaziland, South Africa, Guinea-Bissau, and Kenya. The detailed review has been published elsewhere (Patel, 1995a) and only an overview of the main findings are presented here.

Virtually all the cultures reviewed differentiated between the mind and the body, and the concepts relating to the mind were shared to some extent by the different cultures. The existence of TMPs who specialised in the management of mental illness (Gelfand, Mavi, Drummond, & Ndemera, 1985; Good, 1987; Odejide, Olatawura, Sanda, & Oyenye, 1977; Staugard, 1985) was further evidence of a mind–body differentiation. There were some similarities to Euro-American concepts, evidenced by reports of a "goodness-of-fit" between the two systems' identification of mental illness, and the attempts by some authors to compare traditional concepts about the parts of man to Euro-American concepts, such as Freudian theories about the personality (Mutambirwa, 1989). What differed were the semantics used to describe the mind and concepts relating to its function and localisation. Illnesses of the "spirit" and of the "soul" were probably analogous to mental illness. Although there was some variation about the somatic positioning of the mind, it was mostly localised in the head, chest, and abdominal regions. As Ebigbo (1986) states, this localisation of the mind to somatic structures may explain the phenomenon of somatic presentations of nonpsychotic mental illnesses. Thus, what was perceived by European patients as being palpitations associated with anxiety due to "stress" and worries in the mind, may be perceived by an African patient as palpitations due to imbalance in the function of the heart.

A number of common threads could be identified in the diversity of taxonomies and aetiological models. First, although there was a common assumption that classification was solely on aetiological grounds, there was evidence that phenomenological classifications were also important. Thus, the type and severity of behavioural disturbance was often used to classify broad categories of mental illness; it was within these categories that aetiological models were used for further classification. Second, the classifications used were flexible and patient dependent; thus, even though phenomenology was used by a healer to understand the nature of the illness, an aetiological model was almost always provided since it gave the illness experience meaning for the patient. Third, there was a general classification of illness into the two categories of "natural" and "unnatural" illness; these have clear implications on health service utilisation, since the former category was perceived as being related to physical or environmental causes and could be equally well treated by both biomedical and traditional methods, whereas the latter was seen to be related to traditional beliefs of misfortune and illness and was more likely to be brought to TMPs. Fourth, the role of supernatural factors was prominent in the causation of illness. Though witchcraft is outlawed in most of Sub-Saharan Africa, this category continued to be used as an important way of explaining misfortune. Finally, there was growing evidence that with the influence of colonisation and urbanisation, views about illness were also changing. For example, a study with psychiatric outpatients in Nigeria found that less than half the patients held a supernatural cause as the source of their problem; neurotic illness was more likely to be ascribed to supernatural causes than psychotic illness (Ilechukwu, 1988). Similarly, the diminishing importance of supernatural causal models in urban settings was noted by Good in Kenya (1987).

The review suggested that, most commonly, EMs of mental illnesses in Africa equated them with the biomedical construct of psychotic disorders. Thus, in many studies, when healers or key informants were asked open questions to describe mental illness, they most often described behavioural features related to psychotic illness (Ugorji & Ofem, 1976). It was only when there was more detailed inquiry or the presentation of case vignettes that the extended ramifications of the concepts and classification of mental illness which included neurotic-like disorders were elicited. Kortmann's (1987) finding that, although there existed a general and "neutral" Amharic term to denote mental illness in Ethiopia this excluded many less severe forms of psychiatric disturbance which were not considered as being illnesses, has echoes in studies from other African cultures. Similarly, when case vignettes of different presentations of mental disorder were presented to community samples or primary health care staff, neurotic disorders were rarely viewed as being psychiatric problems (Abiodun, 1991; Erinosho & Ayonrinde, 1978). Indeed, the view that TMPs may not be able to distinguish neurotic and psychotic disorders (Gelfand, 1967) may be largely due to the fact that they do not recognise the former as being related to the latter.

There was a striking similarity in the behavioural symptoms of acute psychotic disorder across cultures, with some behaviours such as aggression being particularly common. Although such patients would be identified as suffering from a psychotic illness by etic criteria, there was much less emphasis on cognitive features such as delusions which are central to psychiatric diagnosis. Neurotic disorders, although often not perceived to be mental disorders, were still recognised by local communities and TMPs as being sources of illness and misfortune. Somatic features predominated, and there were some symptoms that were reported to be particularly common, such as the sensation of crawling under the skin and uncomfortable sensations originating in the region of the heart and abdomen. A number of cognitive features were also identified, though they were often less emphasised. These included fearful feelings, thinking too much, and the mind going blank. Finally, there were several phenomena that bore close similarity to anxiety and depression, such as insomnia, palpitations, and headache. Even though, in general, no distinctions were made between the various categories of neurotic disorder, some studies involving detailed questioning of TMPs uncovered sub-categories which bore similarities to dissociative and panic disorders. Obsessive–compulsive disorders and phobias were rarely recognised.

THE STUDY SETTING

The studies described in this monograph were conducted in Harare, the capital city of Zimbabwe. Zimbabwe is a landlocked nation in south central Africa. She gained independence from colonial rule after a bitter liberation war in 1980. In the 1992 census, Zimbabwe's population was recorded to be just over 10 million (Central Statistical Office, 1995). Just under 70% of the population lived in the rural areas. The population was relatively young with 45% aged below 15 years and only 3% aged over 65 years. Of the adult population (i.e. over 15 years of age), 56% were married. Of the adult population, 38% were either students, "home-makers", or were unable to work due to sickness or old age. Of the remainder, 22% were unemployed. Of those in employment, agriculture accounted for 43% of jobs, most of which were in communal farming. Given the highly seasonal nature of agriculture in Zimbabwe and the fact that most farming is subsistence, this occupation does not offer long-term stability or security to most farmers.

The majority of Zimbabwe's people are of African origin (98%). Although the 1992 census does not report the ethnic composition of the African population, it is widely accepted that the Shona tribe are by far the more numerous, particularly in the Harare region. This group is composed of numerous subclans (e.g. Zezuru, Manyika, Karanga), but all speak Shona (with variations in dialects for each subclan). The other major group are the Ndebele who are concentrated in the southwestern regions of the country. Their language has roots in the Zulu language and is linguistically distinct from Shona. A number of other African nationalities are represented in Zimbabwe, particularly in Harare. Many of these immigrants are also conversant in Shona. Thus, Shona is the most commonly spoken language in Harare and was the language used for the studies described in this book. In the non-African population are the whites and Asians. Both communities, in particular the former, are highly influential in terms of their control of private industry and farming land.

Harare is the administrative and commercial capital of Zimbabwe. It was founded about 100 years ago by British settlers, and until independence in 1980 was called Salisbury. It has a population of approximately 1 120 000 inhabitants (Central Statistical Office, 1995). The city's 42 suburbs can be classified into two types: low-density suburbs which, for historical reasons, house the professional and educated classes (now multiracial), and high-density suburbs, which house most of the city's black population. Household size varies from 2.9 in the low-density suburb of Borrowdale to 4.9 in the high-density suburbs of Workington and Mufakose (City of Harare Health Department, 1994). Health service use differs between these two types of suburb; residents of low-density suburbs use private health facilities, while those of high-density suburbs make greater use of public health facilities and TMP. Private general practitioners (GPs) are also playing an increasing role in primary health care in high-density suburbs.

Zimbabwe is a society in transition. It is witnessing an increasing rural to urban migration and a change in the traditional extended family and clan kinship networks (Romme, 1987). Increasing exposure to European and American culture through films and music is evident in the towns and cities and this is identified as a key influence in the breakdown of traditional kinship ties (Bourdillon, 1987). Zimbabwe made impressive progress in health care in the years following independence. The increased funds available through taxes and foreign aid and the government's policy of supporting primary health care led to impressive improvements in health indices; for example, infant mortality rates reduced from 110 per 1000 live births in 1960 to 73 per 1000 in 1986 (Roemer, 1991). These achievements prompted a recent UNICEF report to describe Zimbabwe as a "beacon for progress towards child survival and development in Sub-Saharan Africa" (Lennock, 1994). Since 1990, however, the achievements of post-independence Zimbabwe are under serious threat due to a combination of reasons. The public resources available for investment in the social sector are being reduced due to slow economic growth in the 1980s, overdependence on overseas financial aid, drought, and, since 1991, the budgetary constraints imposed as a result of the implementation of the World Bank Economic Structural Adjustment Programme (ESAP). One key plank of ESAP has been the reduction in government expenditure which led to the introduction of "user fees" for public health services. This policy has been directly blamed for a fall in primary health clinics attendances despite a growing population (Logie & Woodroffe, 1993). It is anecdotally reported that there are increasing numbers of patients now consulting TMPs. A recent community survey has reported an association between relative poverty, nonconsultation for illness, and poorer health outcomes affecting a sizeable proportion of the sample (Winston & Patel, 1995).

MEDICAL PLURALISM IN ZIMBABWE

Health care in Zimbabwe, like most African countries, is provided by both biomedical and traditional health care providers (Ben-Tovim, 1985). Patients are faced with a varied choice of health care practitioners and may consult different practitioners simultaneously or consecutively.

Biomedicine was introduced in Zimbabwe by the missionaries who preceded the colonial settlers. Following colonisation came the doctors who catered largely to the white settler population. This was the first exposure of biomedicine to the country's black people. Biomedical services were dichotomised in public and private health services. Public health care was provided through hospitals and clinics, and were funded either by the missions or the government. Facilities run by the government tended to be segregated on racial grounds while mission hospitals dealt largely with blacks in the rural areas. Private medical practitioners were concentrated in the urban areas and catered almost exclusively to the white population. Many were economically protected through medical insurance schemes (Roemer, 1991). As the government service grew, an increasing need for district- and rural-based doctors was apparent and, by the 1950s, many such posts became unfilled vacancies. Standards of peripheral care dropped further as the central hospitals sucked in more of the health budget in funding high technology medicine. The new medical school, which graduated its first doctors in 1968, had little impact on the shortage of medical manpower since most new graduates stayed in the urban areas or left the country (Mossop & Stratford, 1986). Sadly, even after independence this trend has not changed with many medical and nursing graduates migrating to work in neighbouring Botswana or South Africa for the better wages offered there. Following independence, the government embarked on an ambitious programme to redevelop the peripheral health services and created the new position of the village health worker with a preventive health role. District hospital staffing levels improved with many expatriate doctors, though the situation remained critical with over a third of posts reported to be vacant in 1995. Of Zimbabwe's 1600-odd medical practitioners, over 1000 are concentrated in the two main cities of Harare and Bulawayo. Thus the average doctor patient ratio of 6500 is unrepresentative of the situation in poor urban areas and rural areas. This shortage of manpower is even more acute in the field of psychiatry; thus, the situation at independence with seven psychiatrists, all in urban areas (Hollander, 1986), had barely improved to about a dozen psychiatrists in 1995.

The Ministry of Health and the City of Harare Health Department provide biomedical health care services in Harare. The two main central teaching hospitals are administered by the Ministry of Health and serve as tertiary referral centres for northern Zimbabwe; the local hospitals and primary health care centres are administered by the City of Harare Health Department. Psychiatric services in the public sector are largely concentrated in the central hospitals, each of which houses an acute unit. At the time of the studies described in this book (1993–1995), these units were staffed mainly by expatriate consultant psychiatrists, local psychiatric trainees and interns, nurses, and occupational therapists. The vast majority of patients suffered from a psychotic illness, often with disturbed behaviour. The emphasis of inpatient care was to obtain a psychiatric diagnosis and provide pharmacological treatments; psychotherapeutic approaches were seldom used (Romme, 1987). A study with 67 referrals to a Harare psychiatric unit revealed that many patients had consulted a TMP earlier and most had bypassed biomedical primary care services (Reeler, 1992). The majority (74%) were acutely psychotic with disturbed behaviour. Delays in seeking psychiatric care were not evident for those consulting TMPs.

PHC are run by the City Health Department and are staffed by general nurses. Eleven community psychiatric nurses were posted in different districts. Their work was concentrated on community care of the chronically mentally ill and they would only occasionally see patients with CMD. Medical officers visited clinics twice or thrice weekly to hold clinics. HIV-related disease was the single most important cause of death, accounting for a third of all deaths in the 25–44 year age group. Suicide was the fourth most common cause of death in the 15–24 year age group accounting for 5% of all deaths (City of Harare Health Department, 1994).

Traditional medicine is an important source of health care in modern Zimbabwe. TMP are grouped into two broad categories: the *n'angas* include spirit mediums, diviners and herbalists; and the *profitas*, who belong to one of the many African Christian churches which flourish in the country and use methods which syncretise traditional treatments and Christian beliefs. The latter belong mainly to the Apostolic churches and divine the causes of illness through the the Holy Spirit (as opposed to the ancestral spirits in the case of *n'anga*). The most obvious role of these different TMPs as depicted in much of the cross-cultural literature is that of the "native medicine-man" in which health is defined along biomedical concepts of disease entities. In addition to health care, however, TMPs are also religious consultants, legal advisors, social workers, marriage counsellors, health educators, and family therapists (Cavender, 1991; Ngwenya, 1992; Nyamwaya, 1992; Staugard, 1985). TMPs are relatively well organised; shortly after independence in 1980, the Zimbabwe National Association of Traditional Healers (ZINATHA) was formed by amalgamating eight other small organisations, with aims not dissimilar to professional bodies representing biomedical practitioners. While ZINATHA plays an important role in registering healers and publishes occasional papers, its role in research and training is limited due to a shortage of trained research staff, financial constraints, and political problems (Chavunduka, 1986). Although maintaining registers of TMPs is an important function of these organisations, it is generally thought that less than half of the 40 000 TMP in Zimbabwe are registered with the ZINATHA (Chavunduka, 1994).

A recent community survey of TMPs was conducted in two suburbs of Harare which were to be the focal points for much of the research described in this book (Winston, Patel, Musonza, & Nyathi, 1995). By means of a multistage tracing procedure, 189 TMPs were identified in the two high-density suburbs of Dzivarasekwa and Mufakose. By contrast, the suburbs were served by 58 primary care nurses and 5 private doctors, which represented a ratio of 3 TMPs per biomedical practitioner. A stratified sample of 110 TMPs were invited for a detailed interview. It was noted that 46% of the final census of TMPs were not registered with a TMP association. None of the *profita* were registered, suggesting that the attempts by ZINATHA to include them in their official registers had not met with much success. The registration bias was relevant since *profitas* and *n'angas* constituted different groups of TMP. *Profitas* were younger and better educated, entered practice at a younger age, and had fewer years experience in practice. Virtually all were affiliated to an African church, most commonly the Apostolic Church. The greater age of *n'anga* and their clients (Winston & Patel, 1995) may reflect a change in health care-seeking patterns, from those based on a traditional world view favoured by an older generation of TMP who are preferred by older community members to those rooted within contemporary syncretic Christianity and favoured by younger members of the community. Both groups of TMP shared common characteristics in their practices. The majority were full time and often saw clients in the evenings and at weekends; in doing so, they appeared to offer a practical and convenient service available at times when clients were better able to access them. The average TMP reported seeing only three to four patients daily. *Profita* tended to charge lower fees and reported themselves as busier than *n'anga*, two findings which may be linked. Many TMPs referred patients to clinics. The predominant reason given for referral was physical illness. Many of those interviewed wished for closer relationships with the biomedical sector, either through easier and more personal referral systems or through opportunities to share or transfer care between the traditional and biomedical sectors. The survey concluded that TMPs were numerous, accessible at hours convenient to clients, familiar with a range of problems, aware of current health concerns, and favourably disposed towards biomedical care (Winston et al., 1995).

SUMMARY

The universalist and culturally relativist approaches to cross-cultural psychiatry need to be integrated to produce research which is not only comparable across cultures but also sensitive to the local culture. Such research needs to be linked to practical clinical goals. Integrating ethnographic and epidemiological methods offers the potential of achieving the goal of a culturally sensitive psychiatry. Common mental disorders (CMD) are amongst the most frequent and disabling of human afflictions. CMD include a wide range of distress states, often presenting with nonspecific somatic complaints and having prominent features of anxiety and depression. Epidemiological studies of mental illness in primary care and community settings in Sub-Saharan Africa have shown that mental illness can be identified with psychiatric interviews in about a quarter of attenders at primary care clinics. Ethnographic studies of mental illness have tended to show that, although mental illness is recognised as a distinct entity from physical illness, the concept of mental illness is mostly related to acute and severe behavioural disturbance and often excludes the distress states subsumed under CMD. Supernatural forces such as witchcraft are one of the commonest causal models for CMD.

Zimbabwe is one of the youngest independent nations in Africa. Its people consult both biomedical practitioners and TMP for health problems. Psychiatric services cannot even cope with the demands placed by those with severe mental disorders; thus, CMD are almost entirely seen and managed by primary health workers who are mainly nurses in primary care clinics and TMPs. Research is needed to describe the concepts of CMD, the indigenous models used to describe and explain CMD, the symptoms which best identify CMD, and the prevalence and risk factors of CMD in biomedical and traditional medical attenders. Through the use of culturally sensitive methods, such research may achieve the twin goals of communicating not only with academic researchers but with those who are in the frontline of primary health care in Zimbabwe.

CHAPTER TWO

The studies

OBJECTIVES

The overall objectives of the studies in this book were to obtain a description of CMD in primary care attenders using methods which integrate ethnographic and epidemiological techniques in the study of psychological disorders. The studies aimed to explore the contribution of culture to the presentation, assessment, classification, and risk factors for CMD in primary care in Harare.

The specific objectives were: (1) to describe the concepts of mental illness of carers in community and primary care based settings; (2) to describe the symptoms and explanatory models of patients with conspicuous psychiatric morbidity (i.e. primary care attenders whom their care providers feel have a CMD); (3) to develop an indigenous measure of CMD which could be used as a case finding instrument for future epidemiological investigations; (4) to examine the relationship between indigenous and biomedical models of mental illness; (5) to determine the prevalence, associations, and risk factors of CMD in primary care attenders.

THE ETHNOGRAPHIC STUDY
Aimed to elicit the concepts of mental illness held by primary care providers

Design: Exploratory

Sample: 76 care providers (22 traditional medical practitioners, 9 community psychiatric nurses, 30 village health workers and 15 relatives of psychiatric patients)

Data collection: Focus group discussions

Elicited screening guidelines for primary care attenders with a probable CMD for use in the next study

THE PHENOMENOLOGY STUDY
Aimed to elicit the symptoms and explanatory models of primary care attenders with conspicuous psychiatric morbidity

Design: Cross-sectional survey

Sample: 110 primary care attenders selected by their care providers
(PHC $n = 53$ and TMP $n = 57$)

Data collection: Qualitative and semistructured interviews

Elicited idioms of distress which formed a preliminary version of a measure of psychiatric morbidity, the Shona Symptom Questionnaire, and elicited two common causal models of illness, *kufungisisa* or "thinking too much" and supernatural causation

THE SHONA SYMPTOM QUESTIONNAIRE (SSQ) STUDY
Aimed to develop the final version of the SSQ, to examine the relationship between CMD and two indigenous models of illness causation, and to determine the prevalence of CMD

Design: Cross-sectional survey

Sample: 302 primary care attenders selected by systematic sampling at PHC ($n = 152$) and consecutive attenders at TMP ($n = 150$)

Data collection: Semistructured interviews

Led to the development of a 14-item SSQ for the detection and measurement of non-psychotic psychiatric morbidity, demonstrated a strong association between indigenous causal models of *kufungisisa* and supernatural causation with biomedical models of CMD and a higher prevalence of CMD in TMP attenders

THE CASE-CONTROL STUDY
Aimed to examine the associations and risk factors for CMD

Design: Unmatched case-control

Sample: 199 cases and 197 controls (defined on basis of SSQ score) selected from PHC, TMP and GP attenders

Data collection: Semistructured interviews

Demonstrated associations of CMD with female gender, economic impoverishment and disability, and confirmed the association with both indigenous models of illness causation

FIG. 2.1 An overview of the studies

THE ETHNOGRAPHIC STUDY[1]

Aims

The aims of this study were to describe the concepts of mental illness held by a diverse range of primary care providers in Harare and to define screening criteria for distress states which approximated CMD for use by health care providers to identify cases for the next study.

Sample

Four groups of care providers were recruited: 22 TMPs recruited through TMP key informants; 9 out of 11 community psychiatric nurses (CPN) working in the City of Harare PHCs; 30 of the 36 village health workers (VHW) from the periurban settlement of Epworth; and 15 relatives (REL) of patients attending psychiatric clinics at the Parirenyatwa Hospital in Harare.

Data collection

Focus group discussions (FGD) were selected as the method of data collection. A focus group questionnaire was designed based on clinical experience and previous ethnographic research suggesting that, although mental illness was recognised as a category of illness by the community and TMPs, it was often equated with severe behavioural disturbances akin to psychotic disorders. Since we wished to generate emic data to compare with biomedical concepts of CMD, the FGD were introduced by informing the care providers that the FGD were not referring to severe madness (*kupenga*) alone but any of the illnesses of the spirit/soul (*mweya*) and mind/thinking (*pfungwa*) and to the problems of those patients who presented with illnesses which were not related to a physical illness. The key concepts which were covered in the FGDs were: the meaning of the term mental illness; the site of the "mind" in the body; the functions of the "mind"; the types and causes of mental illness; the effect of mental illness on the sufferer; the impact of mental illness; and the types of health care which were appropriate. After covering these concepts, three case vignettes describing typical cases of CMD were presented.

A 40-year-old woman with depression and suicidal ideas. For a few months, a 40-year-old woman has been looking very sad, miserable, and

---

[1] See Patel, Musara, Maramba, and Butau (1995a).

unable to look after her home and children, slow in speech and movements. She says that life is not worth living. Nothing seems capable of cheering her up. She does not eat or sleep well and lies on a bed for days without doing anything. Once she even tried to take her own life.

A 34-year-old man with panic attacks and agoraphobia. A 34-year-old man has been unable to use public transport for the past month because he feels unwell and frightened to do so. He used to go shopping with his wife but now feels uncomfortable in markets. Crowds make him break out in a sweat and he feels tense and panicky. When this happens, he feels like something terrible is going to happen and now he spends much time indoors.

A 38-year-old woman with multiple unexplained somatic symptoms. A 38-year-old woman has been complaining of body aches and pains, especially headaches, crawling sensations in her skin, chest discomfort, tiredness, and backache. Physical tests and examinations do not show any sign of a physical illness.

Groups were asked to consider for each vignette the following: what, if anything, was the problem in this case; what were the causes of this problem; what should the person do about it?

Focus group procedure

A total of nine FGD were held with an average of seven to nine participants. The composition of each FGD was determined by the type of carer concerned; thus, groups consisted of TMP or REL or CPN or VHW. The three FGD with VHW were conducted outdoors on a large monolithic rock in Epworth which was the site of their regular meetings. Two of the three FGD with TMP were conducted in the homes of TMP while the third was in the medical school. The remaining FGD (one with CPN and two with REL) were conducted in the medical school. All FGD were conducted by persons familiar to the carer group; thus, the FGD with TMP were conducted by a TMP; the FGD with the VHW were conducted by a nurse who was involved in coordinating their activities as part of the medical school Family Health Programme; the FGD with CPN and REL was conducted by a psychiatric nurse. All FGD were in Shona.

Data analysis

The author was present at all FGD and recorded the proceedings on tapes; these were later transcribed and translated to English for further analysis. Data analysis was done separately for the four carer groups. Analysis involved examining the data for themes and categories which were related to the questions posed. Themes which recurred across FGDs were of special interest because they were potentially more representative. After ordering data according to the questions posed, data were categorised based on responses with similar characteristics and possible associations between data were explored (Varkevisser, Pathmanathan, & Brownlee, 1991).

Link to next study

A series of guidelines which could serve as screening criteria for CMD were drawn up using material from the FGD. Thus, persons with a CMD could include:

1. Patients complaining directly of mental illness categories, such as madness or *kupenga* and thinking too much or *kufungisisa*.
2. Those with illnesses which may be related to mental illness, such as *muroyi* or witchcraft.
3. Those with specific causes of mental illness such as *mbanje* or cannabis and alcohol abuse and head injuries.
4. Those with relationship problems such as marital and sexual problems.
5. Those with social problems and life events such as unemployment and bereavement.
6. Those with illnesses that were perceived to arise either in the head (*musoro*) or the heart (*moyo*).
7. Those with typical psychiatric presentations including: expressions of sadness, tearfulness or suicidal ideas; fear, apprehension or constant worrying; unexplained multiple physical symptoms; acute attacks of fear with physical symptoms such as a rapid heart beat.

THE PHENOMENOLOGY STUDY[2]

Aims

The aim of this study was to record the symptoms and explanatory models of primary care attenders who were considered to suffer from a mental illness by care providers ("conspicuous psychiatric morbidity"). An additional objective was to translate and field test the Revised Clinical Interview Schedule, a standardised psychiatric interview

---

[2] See Patel, Gwanzura, Simunyu, Lloyd, and Mann (1995d).

Study design

Cross-sectional survey of primary care attenders with conspicuous psychiatric morbidity.

Site

Three PHCs in three suburbs and four TMPs selected on recommendation from key informants (including the district TMP organisation secretary) on the basis that these TMPs were locally well known and had sufficient patients to allow the research to be completed within the limited time available. The four TMPs included three *n'angas* and one *profita*.

Sample

The care providers were asked to select patients from consecutive outpatient attenders who had consulted them for illnesses which they thought were presentations of a mental illness. The care providers used both their clinical judgment and the screening guidelines from the Ethnographic Study in the selection of patients.

Instruments

Two instruments were used: the Explanatory Model Interview (EMI) and the Revised Clinical Interview Schedule (CISR).

EMI. This is a semistructured interview developed to elicit explanatory models of illness which incorporates qualitative and quantitative items. The EMI used in this study was an adapted version of the Short Explanatory Model Interview (Lloyd et al., 1996) which, in turn, is based on Kleinman's (1980) suggested questions for eliciting explanatory models:

- What do you call your problem?
- What name does it have?
- What do you think has caused your problem?
- Why do you think it started when it did?
- What does your sickness do to you?
- How severe is it? What do you fear most about your sickness?
- What are the chief difficulties your sickness has caused for you?

Few problems arose in the translation of the EMI to Shona since most of the questions contained no emotional or psychological terms. Indeed, the open nature of the questions meant that the first back translation from the Shona version resulted in a version conceptually similar to the original interview. With advice from a team of bilingual indigenous professionals (including two nurses and a medical anthropologist), some items were adapted: for example, the item about perceived origin of illness (i.e. whether a person felt their distress had an emotional component) was adapted since the closest conceptual equivalent to "emotional" would apply to distress which affected both the "mind" (*pfungwa*) as well as the "soul" (*mweya*) (Mutambirwa, 1989).

A further seven closed items regarding causal models were added after piloting because it was apparent that many patients gave "don't know" responses to open questions about perceived causes. This was, in part, due to embarrassment caused by stating supernatural or nonmedical causes to an interviewer who was from a medical background. Seven causal models were used for the closed questions, which were to be asked after the open question. These causes were based on those elicited in earlier studies on indigenous views of causes of mental disorder (Chavunduka, 1978; Gelfand, 1967): (1) *mudzimu, ngozi, mashave* (i.e. ancestral spirits, aggrieved spirits, and alien spirits, respectively); (2) *muroyi* (witchcraft); (3) *mamhepo* ("bad airs", occasionally related to witchcraft); (4) *mbanje* (cannabis); (5) alcohol; (6) *nhaka* (refers to heredity, but may imply a spiritual inheritance); (7) *kufungisisa* or thinking too much.

The Revised Clinical Interview Schedule (CISR). This is a revised version of a standardised interview developed for clinical evaluation of mental state by Goldberg and colleagues (1970). The CISR is semi-structured interview that can be used by lay interviewers in community and primary care studies of CMD (Lewis, Pelosi, Araya, & Dunn, 1992). The interview is composed of 14 key areas corresponding to major components of nonpsychotic mental disorders as recognised by biomedical psychiatry: somatic symptoms, fatigue, concentration, sleep problems, worry about physical health, irritability, worry, depression, depressive ideas, anxiety, panic, phobias, obsessions, and compulsions. Each key area contains one or two mandatory questions which determine whether the particular symptom group was experienced in the previous week; if the patient responds positively to the mandatory question, a series of scoring questions rates the severity of the symptoms in the previous week leading to a key area score. The total of 14 key area scores comprises the total score (range 0–57) which is a measure of the severity of nonpsychotic psychiatric morbidity. A cut-off score of 11–12 has been validated to determine caseness (Lewis et al., 1992). This was the first time the CISR was used in Zimbabwe.

The Shona version of the CISR was prepared through a series of stages beginning with translation into Shona by two bilingual mental health professionals (a psychiatric nurse and a psychiatrist). The two Shona versions were presented to a third bilingual mental health professional (a psychiatric nurse) for back translation. Based on this back translation, items from either version with the closest semantic equivalence to the original text were selected. For some items, neither translation was correct and the third translator provided a new version for that item. For some items, both the versions were close to the original and were both retained in the interview as alternatives. The Shona version was now presented to five Shona health professionals (a medical anthropologist, two psychiatric nurses, one sociologist, and one TMP). Simultaneously, it was also presented to a Shona linguist with no previous mental health experience for back translation. Emphasis was now laid on content and technical equivalence. As a result of the opinion of the experts, some items were adapted. For example, the item "phobias while using public transport" was reworded to inquire about fear whilst using "emergency taxis" (a common form of public transport).

Interview procedure

Two bilingual researchers who were psychology graduates conducted interviews under supervision by the author. Both underwent training including role play and interviewing psychiatric patients, and special emphasis was laid on achieving competence with conducting qualitative interviews and the use of open-ended probes. After being selected by the care provider and providing consent, the patient was interviewed by a research worker. The EMI was administered first so that the closed questions of the CISR would not bias the reporting of symptoms.

Data analysis

Shona data was translated to English for analyses. The qualitative data generated from the EMI were converted into numerical codes following the method of stepwise reduction of data to discrete categories (Varkevisser et al., 1991):

1. The first 30 interviews were reviewed by the research team. Qualitative data for each item were collated and broad themes identified; for example, for the item "reasons for consultation", themes were "aches and pains", "other somatic complaint", "supernatural complaint" etc.;
2. These themes were allocated numerical codes and the 30 cases coded independently by two researchers. The interrater reliability of the rating codes was estimated. For items with kappas < 0.7, rating codes were refined and altered (see Table 2.1 for examples of final codes);
3. Emic symptoms were elicited by open-ended probing with the key question "what does your illness do to you? For example, what does

TABLE 2.1
Rating codes for the Shona explanatory model interview

*Reason for consultation**
1. Aches and pains (e.g. headache, stomach ache)
2. Other somatic complaints (e.g. difficulty walking, tiredness)
3. Specific somatic diagnoses (e.g. high BP, diabetes)
4. Autonomic complaints (e.g. palpitations)
5. Behavioural complaints (e.g. sleep and appetite, aggression)
6. Psychological complaints (e.g. thinking too much)
7. Marital/family problems (e.g. beaten by spouse)
8. Socioeconomic problems (e.g. homelessness, hunger)
9. Supernatural/spiritual problems (e.g. *mudzimu*, being bewitched)
10. Not applicable/missing

Worries and difficulties caused by illness
1. Ability to care for children/family
2. Ability to maintain or get employment
3. Marital difficulties (e.g. worry that illness may prevent marriage)
4. Difficulties in other relationships (e.g. with in-laws, neighbours)
5. Economic difficulties (e.g. homeless, hungry)
6. Worry about symptoms/outcome of illness
7. Supernatural worry (e.g. bewitched)
8. Other difficulties
9. Not particularly worried/no specific difficulties
10. Missing/not applicable

* Similar facets were used for items on name of illness, cause of illness, and reason for timing.

it do to your body and mind?". Items were enumerated and those which occurred in at least five cases were allocated independent codes. These items were coded dichotomously (not reported/ reported) for the entire sample.

Links to the next study

The Phenomenology Study was linked to the next stage by the idioms elicited from patients which went on to form the preliminary version of an indigenous measure of CMD, the Shona Symptom Questionnaire (SSQ). Two causal models and labels for CMD were elicited frequently from patients in this study, viz., *kufungisisa* and supernatural problems, particularly in relation to witchcraft. The relationship of both these causal models and CMD were to be examined in subsequent studies.

The CISR was found to have reasonable criterion validity in this setting. Nearly 75% of patients with conspicuous psychiatric morbidity were rated as cases on the interview. Some of the CISR items were reworded following the experiences of the interviewers who reported problems with the patients' understanding of these items. The items needed to be adapted or reworded for different reasons. For example, the mandatory question on obsessions was often confused with "thinking too much"; in order to distinguish the two, stress was laid on the distinction between the two concepts by giving examples of obsessional ideas. The Shona translation of some words needed to be adapted; for example the literal translation of "concentration" could not be understood by many patients while the same meaning was adequately conveyed by a Shona word whose back translation to English was "comprehension". Finally, some questions needed two versions since either could convey the same meaning in case of difficulties in understanding one translation, for example a question on hopelessness. Interrater reliability of the Shona CISR was estimated by the method of observer co-ratings, one research worker interviewing the patient and scoring the CISR, the other research worker independently scoring the CISR. In this way 46 patients in the sample were co-rated. Kappa values for individual items ranged from 0.58 to 1.00 (average 0.79). The lower kappas were for the last three key areas of the interview, viz., phobias, obsessions, and compulsions which were recorded infrequently.

THE SHONA SYMPTOM QUESTIONNAIRE STUDY[3]

Aims

The overall objective of this study was to develop the Shona Symptom Questionnaire, to estimate the prevalence of CMD in TMP and PHC attenders and to examine the association between two indigenous constructs, viz. *kufungisisa* and supernatural causation with biomedical constructs of CMD.

Study design

A cross-sectional survey of primary care attenders was undertaken.

Site

The study site was two suburbs in western Harare, Dzivarasekwa and Mufakose. These suburbs were allocated to the study by the City of Harare Health Department. Each suburb was served by a single PHC managed by the City Health Department and staffed by nurses (26 in Dzivarasekwa and 32 in Mufakose). All the nurses worked primarily as

---

[3] See Patel et al. (1997b).

general medical nurses, though each clinic also had one CPN. Dzivar-asekwa had two private general practitioners and Mufakose three; neither suburb had a pharmacist. A cross-sectional community survey in two suburbs (carried out by a team including the author) identified a total of 189 TMPs (Winston et al., 1995) of whom 35 were *profita*. Ten TMPs (five *n'anga* and five *profita*) were randomly selected from a subsample of all the TMPs in the two suburbs who were consulted by at least five patients a day ($n = 21$).

Sample size estimation

The sample size was estimated by power calculations (using the EPI6 software) based on the hypothesis that the causal model of *kufungisisa* was associated with the presence of CMD in this population. This hypothesis was based on studies both by the author and other researchers (Abas, Broadhead, Mbape, & Khumalo-Sakatukwa, 1994) which had suggested that this causal explanation was closely related to CMD. The phenomenology study showed that about 80% of patients with conspicuous psychiatric morbidity stated that their problem had been caused by *kufungisisa*. The hypothesis was that this causal model was more associated with cases of CMD as compared to noncases in the attender population. It was hypothesised that the prevalence of this causal explanation was 80% in the cases as compared to 60% in noncases; power calculations estimated that the minimum sample sizes needed to demonstrate this hypothesis were 89 cases and 178 noncases (95% confidence and 90% power assuming that the ratio of noncases to cases was 2:1).

Sampling

PHC patients were recruited by systematic sampling of consecutive attenders to the clinic (ratio 1:4). The exclusion criteria were: (1) patients attending the antenatal clinic; (2) patients under the age of 16 or over 65 years; (3) patients suffering from an acute medical illness.

If a patient was excluded for any of the above reasons, the next patient in the queue was approached. Sampling in the PHC took place on consecutive weekdays over a period of a month. On average, seven or eight patients were recruited daily.

As there were fewer daily attenders at individual TMP clinics, all consecutive attenders became potential recruits. None of the TMP attenders were consulting for antenatal purposes nor did patients with acute medical emergencies consult TMPs. Thus the only exclusion criterion that applied to TMP attenders was being under the age of 16 or over 65 years. Sampling periods at individual TMPs varied on the basis of numbers of patients recruited from each TMP and the times at which the individual TMP was available for consultation. In all, sampling lasted six weeks and included weekends and evenings (in lieu of two weekdays) when attendances were highest. On average, five patients were recruited daily.

Instruments

The preliminary version of the Shona Symptom Questionnaire (SSQ). Shona idioms of distress elicited in the Phenomenology Study were collated. Altogether, 41 phenomena were reported by at least five patients in the sample. The actual idiom for each type of complaint was identified from the original interview data. In the case of six phenomena, two idioms were commonly used to describe them, so both were included in the questionnaire. These six phenomena were: gait problems/difficulty walking, abdominal ache/pain in the navel region, side ache/*mabayo* (a specific type of pricking side pain), being easily startled/feeling panicky, losing interest in speaking to others/losing interest in things one cared about or enjoyed, and feelings of hopelessness/suicidal ideas. The questionnaire was designed to be administered by a lay interviewer to patients with any level of literacy. Emphasis was placed on simple and clear wording. Questions asked about the presence of symptoms during the previous week: patients were required to respond yes (score 1) or no (score 0). This form of scoring is common in psychiatric screening questionnaires, for example the SRQ. The sum of the question scores was hypothesised to reflect the severity of psychiatric morbidity.

The SSQ was then presented to five bilingual mental health and primary health care professionals to assess the clarity of the wording and to check the face validity of the items. Specifically, they were asked if the instrument appeared to be measuring mental illness and whether it covered all the relevant domains. All items were seen to be relevant in the context that this was a preliminary questionnaire which was to be more thoroughly evaluated in the SSQ Study. The questionnaire was then piloted with 95 participants including community residents, PHC, and TMP attenders. The wording was found to be clear. As a result of piloting, an item on seizures was dropped due to its rarity and the one item on gait problems was dropped due to its similarity to another item.

Many researchers who have developed culturally sensitive measures of psychiatric disorder have recognised the importance of established psychiatric measures in developing new instruments and combined such items with those derived with emic techniques. Cheng and Williams (1986) state in relation to the development of the Chinese Health Questionnaire, "it is foolish to ignore a large body of developmental work." Following the same principles, items from the SRQ (Harding et al., 1980) were added to the 45-item preliminary SSQ. The SRQ is the most commonly used case finding instrument in Africa and the Shona version had been previously used in Zimbabwe (Hall & Williams, 1987; Reeler et al., 1993). The SRQ items were adapted to fit in with the format of the preliminary SSQ, i.e. they were reworded to ask about symptoms in the previous week. It was noted that 9 of the 20 items of the SRQ were conceptually and semantically similar to items on the preliminary SSQ and were assumed to be the same. Thus, an additional 11 items were added. Four items on positive mental health derived from the Shona version of the WHO Quality of Life Interview (Kuyken, Orley, Hudelson, & Sartorius, 1994) were randomly distributed in the preliminary SSQ. These were included to generate a score of positive mental health to examine its relationship with SSQ scores and to detect any yea-saying bias. Thus the version of the SSQ used in this study consisted of 60 items from three sources (see Appendix 1).

The Explanatory Model Interview (EMI). An abridged version of this semistructured interview was used. The following items were included: (1) reasons for consultation; (2) the name or label the patient gave to their illness experience; (3) onset of illness; (4) the patient's view of the source of his/her illness, i.e. whether the illness was purely somatic (arising from the *muviri* or body) or also involved the mind (*pfungwa*) or soul (*mweya*); (5) the patients' view on whether *kufungisisa* had caused their illness; (6) the patients' view on whether supernatural factors such as witchcraft had caused their illness. The last two questions were closed with a dichotomous (yes/no or don't know) response format. The rating codes for the first two items were reduced from those of the original version described in Table 2.1. The new rating codes were: somatic (including codes 1–4 in Table 2.1); psychosocial (including codes 5–8 in Table 2.1); spiritual/supernatural; not applicable/missing.

The care provider judgment. For each patient recruited in this study, the care provider (PHC nurse or TMP) who had been consulted was interviewed with a question adapted from the health staff rating schedule used in WHO studies in primary care (Harding et al., 1980), viz., whether the patient's presenting illness was mainly a physical illness, mainly an emotional or mental illness, or a mixture of both.

Interview procedure

Two interviewers participated in the field work. Both were psychology graduates who were bilingual in Shona and English. Their training included role play and pilot interviews with the interview schedules. Both interviewers had earlier participated in the Phenomenology Study and were proficient in the use of the CISR and EMI. After obtaining consent, each patient was seen by the respective care provider and then directed to the interviewers. One interviewer would elicit the preliminary SSQ data, while the second interviewer (blind to the interviewer 1 data) would use the CISR and interview the care provider. The two sets of interviews were given in a random order.

Case criteria

In the absence of "gold standards" to determine psychiatric caseness, the choice of validating criteria is a difficult and controversial issue. In this study two sets of validation criteria for the SSQ were considered:

1. Etic or biomedical criteria: the Revised Clinical Interview Schedule (CISR) with a cut-off of 11–12 as one which discriminates cases best.
2. Emic criteria: The clinical judgment of the care provider (a rating of whether the patient suffered from an emotional or mental illness, though not necessarily excluding a coexisting physical illness).

While the etic criterion offered the advantage of standardisation and reliability, there was a potential risk of imposing a category fallacy. The latter limitation was unlikely to be significant since the Phenomenology Study had shown that the CISR had satisfactory criterion validity. While the emic criterion offered the advantage of providing an indigenous measure of caseness, there was the problem of the lack of standardisation. Since the aim of the SSQ was to measure psychiatric morbidity, it was felt that the criterion of caseness had to be robust, and given the limitations of both the etic and emic criteria alone and the need to be able to relate emic and etic models of illness, it was decided to define the "gold standard" case criterion as those participants who scored 12 or more on the CISR and whom the care provider judged had a mental illness.

In addition to the above criteria, the criterion of patients' assessment of the emotional origin of illness, as elicited from the EMI data, was also used as a "self-assessed" criterion of caseness.

Data analysis

The statistical procedure used to determine the items of the preliminary SSQ which best discriminated for mental disorder was discriminant analysis with the gold standard case criterion as the outcome. Two preliminary statistical steps were used to reduce the number of items to enter into a stepwise model for discrimination. First, the chi-squared statistic for 56 items of the instrument (excluding the 4 positive mental health items) comparing cases and noncases were determined. From the 56 items, 30 items with the highest chi-squared values (ranging from a value of 18 to 61, $P < .001$) differentiating the two groups of participants were selected. Next, all 56 items were entered into a logistic regression model together; those items with odds ratios > 1 and a significance of at least 0.25 were also selected; all but two of these items were already represented in the 30 items selected using chi-squared tests. Thus a total of 32 items (Appendix 2) were selected for further analysis. These 32 items were then entered into a stepwise forward discriminant analysis. The items selected by this statistical procedure went on to form the final version of the SSQ.

The item scores of the SSQ items were summed to generate an SSQ score for each patient. The psychometric properties of the SSQ were then evaluated in the following ways: by comparing the mean scores for cases and noncases according to different case criteria; by calculating specificity, sensitivity, positive and negative predictive values, and misclassification rates of different cut-off scores with the gold standard as the case criterion to estimate the optimal cut-off score for caseness; by plotting receiver operating characteristics (ROC) curves and computing the area under the curve as an estimate of the overall discriminating power of the SSQ; by comparing SSQ scores with patient self-assessment of the emotional origin of their illness experience as a measure of convergent validity; by comparing SSQ scores with those of the positive mental health items (both individual items as well as the sum total of the four items) as a measure of a divergent validity; and by computing the intraclass correlation coefficient (Cronbach's alpha) and Guttmann's split-half reliability as a measure of the internal consistency of the questionnaire.

Link to the next study

The SSQ Study led to the development of a 14-item questionnaire with satisfactory discriminating ability for identifying probable cases of CMD. Its psychometric properies revealed a high divergent and convergent validity and internal consistency. Validity coefficients showed optimal sensitivity and specificity for case detection at a cut-off score of 7–8, i.e. participants who scored 8 or more were probable cases of CMD. The SSQ was then used in the final study as a case detection measure.

THE CASE–CONTROL STUDY[4]

Aims

The objective of this study was to examine the risk factors and associations of CMD. The variables to be studied were sociodemographic,

---

[4] See Patel et al. (1997c).

economic, life events, alcohol use, disability, and clinical presentation including the patient's beliefs on *kufungisisa* and witchcraft and care provider diagnostic and treatment prescription behaviour.

Site

The study took place in the same two high density suburbs as the SSQ Study, Dzivarasekwa and Mufakose. Both the PHCs in the two suburbs, 4 out of 6 GPs and 14 out of 189 TMPs in the two suburbs participated. The TMPs were selected randomly from a sampling frame of TMPs in the two suburbs who reported at least five consultations a day (Winston et al., 1995).

Sample

Potential participants for inclusion in the study were chosen by systematic sampling of consecutive attenders. The sampling ratios differed at the three care provider sites due to the varying numbers of daily attenders at each site; thus, daily attenders were highest at PHCs where the sampling ratio was 1:4, while the sampling ratio at GP was 1:2. Since the average number of daily attenders at TMP was only five, all TMP attenders were recruited. Patients were included in this study if they were aged between 16 and 65 years; they were excluded if they were temporary visitors to Harare and thus unlikely to be available for follow-up interviews or if they had an acute medical illness requiring immediate hospital referral. All eligible patients selected were given full information about the study and only those who gave written consent for the study and follow-up were selected.

Definition of caseness

All consenting patients were interviewed with the psychiatric screening measure, the Shona Symptom Questionnaire (SSQ). Those who scored 8 or more on the SSQ were classified as likely "cases" while those who scored 7 or less were likely "noncases" or the controls.

Instruments

A list of variables collected from each subject is presented in Appendix 3.

Clinical presentations and explanatory models. This interview elicited data on onset, presenting complaints, patient causal models and whether the patient believed that *kufungisisa* or witchcraft had caused their illness.

Sociodemographic interview. This interview elicited sociodemographic, family, and economic data.

Life event rating scale. This instrument was adapted from the Social Readjustment Scale used in earlier studies in Zimbabwe (Myambo, 1990). A series of life events were inquired about in the previous 12 months. If the patient reported a particular event, the interviewer would probe to determine the emotional response to that event, viz., whether the event was perceived as being stressful or not.

AUDIT. The Shona version of the Alcohol Use Disorders Identification Test, a 10-item questionnaire developed in a multinational collaborative study by the WHO (Babor & Grant, 1992; Babor, de la Fuente, Saunders, & Grant, 1992), was used for this study. Scoring guidelines recommend that scores of 8 or more have the highest sensitivity for hazardous consumption and/or recurrent intoxication.

Disability. This interview began with an open question probing the way the illness had affected the patient's life. Next, the Brief Disability Questionnaire (BDQ) (Von Korff et al., 1996), a Shona version of which had been previously used in a WHO study on somatoform disorders, was used. This questionnaire generates a total score of disability (range 0–22) plus two questions on the number of days in the previous month in which the patient was unable to do his or her regular work and was bedridden as a result of the illness. The final component was a three-point continuous measure of the patients' perception of their overall quality of life adapted from the Shona version of the WHO Quality Of Life interview (Kuyken et al., 1994).

Care provider assessment data. PHC staff and GPs were asked to complete a clinical data sheet on each patient in the study which recorded the current diagnosis and current oral and injectable treatment. TMP were interviewed for each of their patients to ascertain diagnosis and cause of illness and their view on the role of ancestral spirits, witchcraft, and *kufungisisa* in the illness.

Interview procedure

A team of four interviewers were involved in the field work. All were indigenous Zimbabweans, fluent in Shona and English, and from a social science or psychology background. Rigorous training in the use of the interview schedule included role play and pilot interviews with psychiatric outpatients. Practice sessions continued until satisfactory interrater reliability was achieved (kappas for quantitative items > 0.7). The interviewers were in the field for a period of two months, one month in each of the two suburbs, and worked concurrently in the different care provider sites. Screening with the SSQ took place while patients waited to see the care provider, while the main interview was randomly carried out either before or after the consultation.

Data analysis

Key sociodemographic and clinical variables were compared between the samples recruited from the three care provider sites. Data were then analysed in terms of the study design, i.e. comparing cases with noncases. Chi-squared tests (with Yates correction) were calculated for categorical variables. T tests and Mann–Whitney U tests were computed for parametric and nonparametric continuous variables respectively. Where appropriate, simple odds ratios were computed as well as odds ratios adjusted for sex, age and site of recruitment.

CHAPTER THREE

Results of the studies

CONCEPTS OF MENTAL ILLNESS OF PRIMARY CARE PROVIDERS

This section describes data from the Ethnographic Study.

The sample

Altogether 9 focus group discussions (FGD) were conducted involving a total of 76 care providers. The demographic characteristics of the participants were:

1. Village health workers ($n = 30$); age mean 46.9 years; *SD* 8.2 years. Sex: females = 26; males = 4; years of experience: mean 8.1 years; *SD* 1.1 years.
2. Traditional medical practitioners ($n = 22$); *n'anga* ($n = 16$) and *profita* ($n = 6$). Age mean 47.4 years; *SD* 12.7 years. Sex: females = 15; males = 7; years of experience: mean 17.2 years; *SD* 19.1 years (range 6 months to 71 years).
3. Community psychiatric nurses ($n = 9$): age mean 37.7 years; *SD* 4.4 years; sex: all female; years of experience: mean 14.3 years; *SD* 3.5 years.
4. Relatives ($n = 15$): age mean 42.3 years; *SD* 7.9 years. Sex: females = 14; males = 1.

Psychiatric diagnoses among the patients: schizophrenia and manic depressive illness.

All the participants spoke Shona. The majority subscribed to one of the many Christian churches in Zimbabwe; the commonest were Methodist (*n* = 17), Salvation Army (*n* = 7), Apostolic (*n* = 11), Anglican (*n* = 9), and Roman Catholic (*n* = 10). Two participants denied any religious affiliation. Other than the nurses, only a handful of care providers were educated beyond the 'O' level stage.

Basic concepts of mental illness

Mental illness was recognised by all care providers as a category of illness in which behavioural changes were characteristic. The person lost his or her ability to reason and to look after the family. The term *kupenga* was frequently used, literally translated as "madness". Such illness was similar to the biomedical concept of acute psychosis. On probing about other illnesses which affected the mind or soul, *kufungisisa*, *mamhepo* (bad airs, often associated with witchcraft) and *pfukwa* or *ngozi* (angry spirits of persons who were killed) were mentioned frequently. CPNs broadly defined mental illness as occurring when a person was behaving in a manner which was unacceptable or contradictory to the norms of the community one lived in.

All the care providers agreed that the mind resided in the head region (*musoro*). Most also pointed to the role of the heart (*moyo*) as being closely connected with the mind. Thus "when someone thinks a lot, the heart becomes heavy" and when someone stole "it is the heart which decides it, and the brains work out how to do it." Similarly, "our thoughts originate from the heart and then move up to the mind" and that "if a person worries a lot, they can experience chest pain." The CPNs all felt that the mind was in the head and the brain, but also commented that they were taught by the elders in the community that the mind resided in the heart.

The principal function of the mind was to organise and plan one's life and that of one's family. The mind determined right from wrong. While "the mind is what makes a person do what they want to do," it also imposed certain socially determined restrictions on behaviour. The mind was the "actual person"; a person without a mind was like a corpse, because he or she could not think. The brain was a broader entity and had many parts with varying functions, such as sensation and movements.

Types and causes of mental illness

CPNs described types and causes of mental illness similar to biomedical nosology, describing categories such as psychoses and depression. When asked about traditional concepts of illness, their views resembled those of the other care providers. The types and causes of mental illness were closely related, the majority of illness being caused by supernatural factors. Supernatural forces could cause misfortune and illness for two reasons, either as a consequence of acts committed by the patient or his family or due to the actions of other persons who used supernatural means to inflict misfortune.

In the first group of supernatural causes, if a person or one of his family broke a social taboo, then spirits would be angered and cause illness. Spirits were of many types, the commonest ones thought to cause severe mental illness being *ngozi* and *pfukwa*. These were the spirits of persons killed either by the patient or by one of his ancestors. *Mudzimu* (family ancestral spirits) and *shave* (alien spirits) could also possess individuals. The former could cause mental illness by abandoning their role of protecting their descendants due to their disrespectful conduct. Such possession needed to be distinguished from that which occurred when the spirits wanted to "come out" through a family member as a sign that he or she was a spirit medium; in these cases, a *n'anga* was consulted and he would clarify that the person was not really mentally ill. Common examples of situations which could lead to illness due to angering of ancestral spirits included:

1. Crimes committed either by the patient or one of his ancestors. These crimes varied from theft to murder and could have occurred several generations earlier. The continuing cycle of illness and misfortune could only be ended if adequate compensation was given to the aggrieved family.
2. Breaking social rituals, e.g. *mombe yeumai* in which a cow was to be given to the bride's mother as *roora* (bride price) or if a deceased person's property was not distributed according to tradition.
3. Acquiring unnecessary charms or amulets or other traditional items for protection or for acquiring wealth and the excess use of "love" potions or *mupfuhwira* (used secretly by a person to make their spouse more affectionate and attentive) could anger the spirits.

Supernatural means could also be used by others, such as relatives, neighbours or friends, or even strangers to inflict illness. The commonest method was through witchcraft (*muroyi*) or sorcery. Witchcraft (which was intrinsic to a person, to his or her soul or personality) was distinguished from sorcery (which was extrinsic and was merely a tool or a technique employed under certain circumstances). These methods were commonly used as a result of someone's jealousy at the success or prosperity of the victim. Witchcraft could cause mental illness in a variety of ways, such as by the use of evil spirits or items such as *zvivanda*, *tokoloshi*, and *zvishiri* (birds or animals used in witchcraft). *Zvidhoma* was a dead person who was raised either to bewitch someone or to seek redress for unresolved grievances. CPNs felt that, in some instances, supernatural explanations helped patients understand why they were suffering and what needed to be done to correct this.

A variety of other causes and types of mental illness were given. Although some accounted for the illness as a direct consequence of the causal factor (such as alcohol damaging the brain), in many instances (such as head injuries following a car accident), a supernatural factor was also sought to answer the fundamental question of *why* the person had a car accident. "Biological" causes of mental illness included head injuries; AIDS; epilepsy; chronic physical illness; drug abuse (especially cannabis); alcohol abuse especially abuse of illicit brews such as *kachasu* or *chikokiyema*; and old age. Children who suffered high fever and convulsions could grow up with mental illness. "Psychological" factors included: thinking too much about problems; bereavement or sickness in close relatives; excessive reading and studying; relationship problems, especially marital conflict and divorce; and loneliness. "Socioeconomic" factors included: poverty; infertility; and unemployment. Many of these causes could also be the result of mental illness. While it was recognised that mental illness ran in some families, the cause was usually the passing on of the spirit of the mentally ill person. Certain specific types of mental illnesses were also described (see Table 3.1).

Symptoms of mental illness

A range of symptoms were described (see Table 3.2). The essential features were behavioural changes and the loss of the ability of self-care. Somatic presentations were partly due to the social stigma attached to mental illness. Sexual complaints were difficult to elicit due to social customs (e.g. the impropriety of young nurses asking older patients such personal questions) and the lack of privacy in crowded primary care clinics. In some patients, symptoms worsened during certain phases of the lunar cycle.

Impact of mental illness

The most important effects were on family relationships. The sexual relationship of a couple could be impaired by an increased or decreased sexual drive. Women could become promiscuous while men could force sex on their wives and become violent if they refused. In trying to determine reasons for the illness, family ties were often disrupted. For example, when a woman became mentally ill, it was often her family which was blamed, leading to quarrels; some care providers remarked that, in this respect, mental illness was similar to AIDS, in which blame was passed around

TABLE 3.1
Shona categories of mental illness described by health care providers

Category of illness	Description/comments	Biomedical equivalent
Kupenga	Severe behavioural disturbance with aggression, inappropriate and disturbed behaviour	Psychosis
Mamhepo	Bizarre behaviour, headaches, sudden mutism, sitting motionless for hours	?Hysteria
Mhengeramumba	Mild variety of mental illness which only manifests in the home	?
Kufungisisa	Thinking too much, excess worry about problems, exams, etc. May appear sad	?Anxiety or depression
Kutanda botso	Acute and brief behavioural disturbance following breaking a major taboo (such as striking parents)	?Brief reactive psychosis
Zvipotswa	Person tries to harm someone by using witchcraft, but fails and becomes mentally ill	?
Kushaya unhu	Person behaves in a manner contradictory to community norms, e.g. is disrespectful	?Antisocial personality
Tsviyo or pfari	Convulsive movements, often associated with behavioural problems	Epilepsy

from husband to wife and so on. Accusations of witchcraft could disrupt family ties. The patient was shunned by others and isolated from the community and often ended up homeless. Since many mental disorders were incurable, there was considerable expense in caring for the patient. The financial burden was increased due to the cost of medication and consultations with private doctors and *n'angas*. The family of the mentally ill person was laughed at and ostracised by others such as neighbours. Relatives could themselves become miserable as a result of these stresses.

Sources of care for the mentally ill

Both biomedical and traditional care providers played a role in the management of mental illness. Hospitals were especially useful for "biological" or "natural" causes such as head injuries and treatment of physical problems such as dehydration. *N'angas* were able to diagnose the real cause of the illness, such as bewitchment, and initiate treatment that would provide a definite and permanent cure. Some relatives felt that *n'angas* helped the patient think more clearly and protected him or her from evil spirits. The treatment could include herbal medicines, steam baths, scarification, or instructions to the patient and family to correct broken taboos or crimes. For example, if someone had become mentally ill because of stealing, he was required to plead with the owner and compensate him for the stolen goods. *Profitas* usually required their

TABLE 3.2
Phenomena of mental disorder described by health care providers

Phenomenon	Types of disturbance and examples
Behavioural	Aggressive: verbal and physical
	Disinhibited: disrobing or urinating in public
	Risky: wandering away from home, running between cars, burning clothes
	Bizarre: eating or smearing faeces, laughing inappropriately, hitting oneself, wearing several layers of clothing, hoarding rubbish
	Agitation and restless behaviour
	Retardation: lying immobile, staring into space
	Sleep: increased or decreased
	Loss of appetite and weight loss
	Sexual: "battery is flat"; "nothing is happening in bed"
Impaired self-care	Not washing, eating dirty food, wearing torn clothes, being unable to look after family
Mood	Irritability
	Sadness
Speech	Increased speed
	Irrelevant nonsensical speech
	Becoming mute
Cognitive	Thinking too much
	Forgetfulness
	Becoming suspicious, e.g. that food is poisoned
Somatic	Headaches, palpitations, weakness, chest pains, infertility in women, high blood pressure, blackouts, gait disturbances.
Perceptual	Hearing voices
	Seeing things others cannot

patients to belong to their church and used a range of treatments including emetic potions, prayer, holy water and biting to remove foreign bodies.

CPNs commented on the particular difficulties of working in busy clinics with little time or privacy to gain the patient's confidence and inquire about personal and family issues which were relevant to their problems. They accepted that many families choose a form of care based on their beliefs regarding the illness and that many families consulted more than one care provider. For example, although the symptoms of a schizophrenic patient were controlled with antipsychotic medication from a clinic, the family would also take him or her to a *n'anga* to perform necessary rituals.

Case 1: A 40-year-old female with depression

All the care providers identified such persons in their community. Some labelled this as *kufungisisa*. Many felt that this was not an "illness" but a reaction to severe life stresses. As one REL said "I do not think this woman is ill . . . she is suffering from worry." Poverty, marital problems such as violence by the husband, bereavement, *kufungisisa*, too many "life problems", illness in the family, laziness, being bewitched, excess of love potions, lack of friends, and not sharing problems with other people were identified as possible causes. The thought of wanting to kill herself could have been inherited from her ancestors, one of whom may have committed suicide. CPNs identified this vignette as depression and commented that such patients often presented with sleep problems or following an overdose, often of antimalarials. Many VHWs felt that she did not need medical treatment but would benefit by socialising in women's clubs or church groups and sharing her problems with friends. Her husband needed education and the family could be helped with their financial problems. *N'angas* could help by getting rid of the evil spirits responsible for the wish to want to kill herself. Some RELs put their trust in biomedical treatments especially those who had suffered similar symptoms and failed to respond to traditional treatment. Visiting a church and talking to a cleric could also be helpful. CPNs said that many patients were taken initially to TMPs and only those who failed to respond consulted at clinics.

Case 2: A 34-year-old male with agoraphobia and panic disorder

Many care providers identified such persons in their community, including some who had fought in the Liberation War and others who had suffered accidents (including one of the VHWs). Road accidents were the most important cause; thus, the patient could imagine that another accident would happen causing him to fear getting in a car. In some cases, the patient or his ancestor may have killed someone in a car accident and did not make amends, leading to possession by the *ngozi* (aggrieved spirit) of the victim. *Kufungisisa*, bereavement, infertility, divorce, physical illness, failures in life, and *mamhepo* were other causes. The patient could be possessed by ancestral spirits who were unaccustomed to cars and the smell of petrol. He could be bewitched by people who were jealous when they saw someone working and doing well. He could have many women friends who gave him love potions. A person with this problem could go for a whole year without leaving his house. Several treatment approaches were advocated: support and reassurance; encouragement to make trips in a car beginning with short distances and gradually increasing it; and being taken by friends to crowded places such as football games and being reassured that there was nothing to fear. Some TMPs said that he should get permission from the spirits before boarding a bus or car. He could also be treated with *bute* (snuff) and rituals such as using a fowl to carry away the aggrieved spirits.

Case 3: A 38-year-old female with unexplained somatic symptoms

Many care providers not only knew such patients but some admitted that they themselves fitted the description. Since the doctors failed to find a cause, some RELs felt that the most likely reason for this woman's problems were to do with her ancestors. Possession by *mudzimu*, laziness, old age affecting muscles and veins, infertility, *kufungisisa*, *mamhepo*, and being bewitched were identified as possible causes. A variety of spiritual treatments used by *n'angas* and *profitas* were appropriate for such patients. CPNs felt the main problem was anxiety and that careful questioning often revealed symptoms typical of psychological distress.

SYMPTOMS AND EXPLANATORY MODELS OF CMD

This section describes data from the Phenomenology Study.

The sample

Primary care providers selected 110 patients from consecutive outpatients on the basis of their clinical assessment that the patient had an emotional disorder (i.e. conspicuous psychiatric morbidity) and 109 completed both the CISR and EMI (1 patient completed the EMI only). Data were analysed for the sample as a whole, and for PHC ($n = 53$) and TMP cases ($n = 57$) separately. The mean age of the sample was 32.5 years (*SD* 11.7, range 15–70). Females comprised 65% of the TMP and 85% of the PHC sample; 57% were living with a partner, 14% were divorced or separated and 4.5% were widowed. 85.5% had not completed school and 82% were not in full-time employment; unskilled work such as selling vegetables was the most common type of employment (7%). Of the sample 80% subscribed to one of many Christian churches operating in the area of which the Apostolic Church had the largest following (24%). The rest of the sample denied any religious affiliation.

Explanatory models

Reasons for consultation. Up to three reasons for consultation were recorded for each patient. The majority of cases presented a somatic complaint, e.g. aches and pains (58%) or stated specific somatic diagnostic labels, e.g. high blood pressure (15%) or a nonspecific somatic complaint, e.g. dizziness (39%). Other reasons stated were psychological (e.g. thinking too much), marital complaints, socioeconomic complaints and supernatural complaints. Supernatural complaints, e.g. "my *mudzimu* has been blocked", were more common in the TMP group (see Table 3.3).

Name of illness. Respondents were asked whether they had a particular name for their illness. Specific somatic diagnostic labels, e.g high blood pressure, were commoner in the PHC group while supernatural labels, e.g. *mamhepo* or being bewitched, were commoner in the TMP group (see Table 3.3). Other labels used were psychological labels such as *kufungisisa*, nonspecific somatic names, e.g. headache, and relationship problems, e.g. infidelity.

Onset of illness. More than half the sample had a chronic illness (>1 year) with 42% suffering more than two years. Acute presentations were commoner amongst PHC attenders while two-thirds of TMP attenders had a chronic illness (Table 3.3).

Parts of body affected. Respondents were asked to name up to three parts of the body which they felt were affected by their illness. The head was quoted by over half the sample. Other parts commonly cited were the

TABLE 3.3
Comparison of explanatory models between TMP and PHC attenders with conspicuous psychiatric morbidity

Variable	PHC (%)	TMP (%)	χ^2 (df = 1) two-tailed P
Reason for consultation			
Supernatural	0	15	5 (Fisher's) < .01
Name of illness			
Somatic	23	3.5	8.8; < .01
Supernatural	7.5	39	13.7; < .001
Onset of illness			
> 1 year	36	66	9.2; < .01
Origin of illness			
Body mainly	24	7	5.7; < .01
Soul mainly	7.5	35	12.2; < .001
Most important cause of illness			
Somatic	17	5	3.9; < .05
Supernatural	9	44	16.4; < .001
Perceived causes			
Mamhepo ("bad airs")	47	67	4.3; < .05
Angry ancestral spirits	32	58	7.4; < .01
Reason for timing of illness			
Somatic	26	5	7; < .01
Supernatural	11	37	9.7; < .01
Prognostic sssessment			
Fatal outcome or suicide if untreated	28	46	4.7; < .05

stomach (47%), the chest or heart (41%), the legs (30%), the back (16%) and the "mind" (8%). About 8% of women cited their reproductive and genital organs.

Mind/body/soul origin.   Respondents were asked whether they felt their illness was one of the body alone or also involved the mind or soul; 85% felt their illness affected their mind or soul. PHC attenders were more likely to perceive their illness as being mainly of somatic origin while TMP attenders were more likely to localise the soul (*mweya* or spirit centre) as the main source of illness (Table 3.3).

Cause of illness.   Up to three possible causes for their illness were recorded. Supernatural causes such as being bewitched and *mamhepo* were mentioned by 45.5% of the sample. Other causes were specific somatic diseases (17%), e.g. venereal disease; socioeconomic causes (19%), e.g. homelessness; psychological causes (18%), e.g. thinking too much; marital causes (19%), e.g. physical abuse by husband; and bereavement (12%). PHC attenders were more likely to identify somatic causes as the "most important cause" while TMP attenders identified supernatural causes more commonly (Table 3.3).

Perceived causes.   *Kufungisisa* was seen as a possible cause by over 80% in both groups while witchcraft was seen as a cause by over 50%. TMP cases were more likely to admit that *mamhepo* and angry ancestral spirits were possible causes (Table 3.3). Alcohol, cannabis, and heredity were rarely seen as potential causes.

Reason for timing.   Supernatural factors (25%); somatic factors, e.g. pregnancy (15%); and marital factors, e.g. separation (21%) were often cited as reasons for the timing of the illness. Somatic factors were more common in the PHC group and supernatural factors in the TMP group (Table 3.3); the latter group comprised mainly patients who ascribed their illness to the actions of a jealous person.

Worries/difficulties caused by the illness.   Respondents were asked to list up to three worries or difficulties. The ability to care for one's family (36%); losing one's job or difficulties gaining employment (45%); marital problems (42%); economic hardships due to impairment of working ability or marital separation (40%); difficulties in other relationships, most often in-laws or neighbours (34%); and worry about the outcome of the illness (36%) were common in both groups.

Seriousness of illness.   In response to this closed question, 75% of the sample saw their illness as being very serious. On the basis of an item on the degree of impairment in the CISR, 65.5% of participants were unable to complete an activity of daily living as a result of their illness.

Prognostic assessment.   A fatal outcome and suicide were reported more frequently by TMP attenders (Table 3.3). Following treatment, over 80% of attenders of both groups expected a complete cure.

Emic phenomenology

Altogether 41 phenomena which were reported by at least 5 subjects were recorded (see Table 3.4). Many phenomena resemble classic etic phenomena associated with CMD, e.g. tiredness and dizziness. Some phenomena have no obvious etic equivalent, such as "veins/nerves pulling"; sensation of things moving around the body; feeling as though "my behaviour has changed"; a complaint of high blood pressure; hot/cold phenomena such as "burning in the feet"; and unusual chest complaints such as "prickling pains in the heart" or "electric shocks in the chest".

Etic phenomenology

The response rates of the key areas of the CISR are reported in Table 3.5. Most key areas were reported by more than half the cases. Panic attacks were moderately common, while obsessions, compulsions and phobias were rare. The intraclass correlation coefficient was high (Cronbach's alpha = 0.86); the highest correlations were between anxiety and panic (Pearson's $r = 0.62$; $P < .001$) and anxiety and depression (Pearson's $r = 0.53$; $P < .001$). Feelings of guilt, worthlessness and hopelessness were reported by 45% to 68%. Suicidal ideas were present in 12%. Autonomic features such as palpitations, sweating hands, nausea, and breathing difficulties were reported by 42% to 68%. According to the recommended cut-off score for caseness (11–12) 73% of the sample were etic cases.

DEVELOPMENT OF THE SHONA SYMPTOM QUESTIONNAIRE (SSQ)

This section presents data from the SSQ Study.

The sample

One patient (from a PHC) refused to participate in the study. A total of 302 participants (PHC = 152; TMP = 150) were recruited. Six were unable to give a precise age (instead, they could only state a general range such as

TABLE 3.4
Emic phenomenology of primary care attenders with conspicuous psychiatric morbidity

---

Aches and pains
  Headache**
  Abdominal ache**
  Chest/heart ache*
  Back ache*

                                                 Leg ache*
                                           "Side" ache (*mabayo*)
                               Other somatic symptoms

  Tiredness*
  Lack of energy*
  Dizziness*
  Blackouts*
  Palpitations*
  Unusual chest sensations, e.g. prickling pains*
  Weight loss*
  Pfari (fits)
  Gait problems
  Hot or cold sensations
  Sensations of something moving in the body
  "High blood pressure"
  Nausea and vomiting
  Abdominal discomfort after meals/bloating
  Difficulty breathing or feeling suffocated
  Sensation of veins and nerves being pulled
  Shaking/trembling
  Excess sweating
Cognitive and perceptual symptoms
  Thinking too much**
  Worry about life's problems*
  Worry about physical health*
  Forgetfulness*
  Irritability*
  Nightmares/disturbing dreams*
  Being easily startled by trivial things
  Sadness
  Lack of concentration
  Not feeling like speaking or being spoken to
  A feeling as if one's behaviour had changed
  Hallucinations
  Suicidal ideas
  Feeling confused or as if one was losing one's mind
Behavioural symptoms
  Sleep disturbances**
  Loss of appetite**
  Tearfulness

**: Phenomena reported by over 50% of the sample. *: Phenomena reported by 25% to 50% of the sample. Rest of phenomena reported by less than 25% of the sample.

TABLE 3.5
Etic phenomenology of primary care attenders with conspicuous psychiatric morbidity

Key areas	%	Number (n = 109)
Depression	85.5	94
Worry	85.5	94
Anxiety	84.5	93
Worry about physical health	83	91
Tiredness/fatigue	77	86
Somatic symptoms (worsened by feeling low, anxious or stressed)	70	77
Sleep disturbances	69	76
Poor concentration/forgetfulness	60	66
Irritability	52	57
Panic attacks	27	30
Compulsions	4.5	5
Obsessions	1	2
Phobias	0	0

"I was born sometime in the 1960s"): the mean age of the rest of the sample was 30.9 years (SD 12.1); there was no difference between the TMP and PHC samples. Two-thirds of the sample (66%) were female. Just under three-quarters (74%) of participants were not in formal employment; 13% were employed in unskilled labouring jobs. More than half the sample were married (57%) and a quarter (24%) were single. A quarter of the sample had completed at least secondary schooling. Just over a quarter (27%) stated that they had no formal religion; the remainder of the sample was mostly Christian (72%) with a small Muslim group (1%). TMP attenders were more likely to be female (73% vs. 58%, OR 1.9, 95% CI 1.2–3.2), to be unemployed (88% vs. 60%, OR 4.9, 95% CI 2.7–8.8) and to be widowed or separated (37% vs. 21%, OR 2, 95% CI 1.1–3.7). After adjusting for all three associations, only being unemployed remained associated with the TMP sample ($P < .001$).

Clinical characteristics and explanatory models

Most patients (90%) presented with somatic complaints, ranging from aches and pains to specific diagnoses such as tuberculosis in patients attending follow-up clinics. The remainder were mostly those seeking help for social or marital reasons, such as conflicts with spouse and hunger. Such reasons for consultations were commoner amongst TMP attenders (19% vs. < 1%; OR 34.6, 95% 4.9–694.9, $P < .001$). TMP attenders were more likely to label their illness experience as being psychosocial, e.g.

poverty or loss of job, or supernatural, e.g. being bewitched (see Table 3.6). Nearly half the participants (49%) had an acute illness (onset less than one month). Nearly half (47%) viewed their illness as being mainly somatic; more than a third (37%) felt the illness involved both body and mind/soul while 46 individuals (15%) felt it mainly involved the mind/soul; 62% felt that *kufungisisa* had caused their illness while 50% felt that supernatural factors had caused their illness. TMP attenders were more likely to have a chronic illness, to feel that their illness had an emotional component, and to believe that supernatural factors had caused their illness (Table 3.6). After adjusting for all statistically significant clinical and explanatory model variables in Table 3.6 and gender and age, chronicity ($P < .001$), supernatural name of illness ($P < .01$) and belief in supernatural causation of illness ($P < .001$) remained associated with being a TMP attender.

Classification of cases and noncases

Two sets of case criteria were initially considered: (1) Biomedical or etic criteria based on the scores on the CISR: 156 of the 302 participants (52%) scored 12 or more on the CISR and were classified as "etic cases"; and (2) Emic criteria based on the clinical assessment of the care provider: 179 (59%) were classified as "emic cases" by care providers.

The relationship between the etic and emic criteria is discussed later. The gold standard of caseness was agreement between the emic and etic criteria on the basis of which 100 participants were classified as cases and the remainder (202) as noncases. All analyses in this section refer to the gold standard case criterion.

TABLE 3.6
Comparison of clinical and explanatory model variables between TMP and PHC attenders

Variable	TMP %	PHC %	Odds ratio (95% CI)	Two-tailed P value
Name of illness				
Psychosocial	27	6	5.9 2.6–13.5	< .001
Name of illness				
Supernatural	18	5	4 1.7–9.7	< .01
Onset				
> 1 month	76	27	8.6 5.1–14.4	< .001
Perceived origin of illness				
Mind/soul involved ($n = 300$)	64	41	2.6 1.6–4.1	< .001
Supernatural causal model	73.5	27	7.4 4.5–12.4	< .001

Symptoms and explanatory models of cases and noncases

Cases were more likely to present with nonsomatic complaints, e.g. supernatural or psychological complaints (13% vs. 8%) and were more likely to label their illness as being a psychosocial one, e.g. poverty or marital conflict (21% vs. 13%). Cases were more likely to have a chronic illness, to consider that their illness also affected their mind/soul, and to consider that supernatural factors and *kufungisisa* had caused their illness (see Table 3.7).

Etic phenomenology

Psychiatric phenomenology was examined from the CISR scores (see Table 3.8). Cases scored higher on all key area scores other than obsessions and compulsions for which there were few positive respondents (three and six, respectively). Depression and anxiety were reported by over 90% of cases while sleep disturbances, worry about physical health, depressive ideas and worries were reported by over 80%.

A principal component analysis with varimax rotation was carried out with 12 CISR key areas (excluding obsessions and compulsions due to low frequency of ratings). This resulted in the extraction of two factors with eigen values > 1. The two factors accounted for 48% of the total variance. An examination of the two factors (see Table 3.9) shows that all key areas other than phobias and panic load maximally on factor 1 which accounted for 39% of the variance. This factor may be described as a "mixed anxiety–depression" factor. Factor 2 which accounts for 9% of the variance has two key areas, phobias and panic, which load maximally. This factor may be described as a "panic–phobia" factor.

TABLE 3.7
Comparison of clinical and explanatory model variables between cases and noncases

Variable	Case %	Noncase %	OR 95% CI	Two tailed P value
Onset				
>1 month	60	47	1.7 1.03–2.7	.03
Perceived origin of illness				
Mind/soul also involved ($n = 300$)	76	43.5	3.0 1.8–5.1	<.001
Supernatural causal model	60	45	1.8 1.1–2.9	<.01
Kufungisisa as a causal model	74	56	2.2 1.3–3.8	<.001

TABLE 3.8
CISR key area responses and scores for cases and noncases

CISR key area	% of positive responses cases/noncases	Mean scores (SD) for cases vs. noncases; Mann–Whitney U test; P value
Somatic symptoms	76/28	2.3 (1.4) vs. 0.8 (1.5); $z = -7.6$; < .001
Fatigue	70/36	2.1 (1.6) vs. 0.9 (1.4); $z = -6.2$; < .001
Concentration	52/19	1.2 (1.3) vs. 0.3 (0.8); $z = -6.2$; < .001
Sleep complaints	81/32	2 (1.4) vs. 0.7 (1.2); $z = -7.8$; < .001
Irritability	52/18	1.3 (1.4) vs. 0.4 (0.9); $z = -6.3$; < .001
Worry about physical health	81/46.5	2.1 (1.3) vs. 1.1 (1.4); $z = -5.6$; < .001
Depression	92/46	2.5 (1.2) vs. 1 (1.3); $z = -8.4$; < .001
Depressive ideas	83/39	2.5 (1.7) vs. 0.8 (1.2); $z = -8.3$; < .001
Worry	84/37	2.7 (1.4) vs. 0.9 (1.4); $z = -8.9$; < .001
Anxiety	93/40	2.9 (1.2) vs. 1 (1.4); $z = -9.4$; < .001
Phobias	16/5	0.3 (0.7) vs. 0.1 (0.4); $z = -3$; < .01
Panic	36/6	0.9 (1.4) vs. 0.2 (0.7); $z = -6.5$; < .001
Compulsions	3/0	not calculable
Obsessions	3/1.5	0.08 (0.5) vs. 0.03 (0.3); $z = -0.89$; $P = .3$

In response to an item on whether the patient's illness had stopped him or her from completing a household or occupational task in the previous week, 68% of cases responded positively as compared to 39% of noncases (OR 3.4, 95% CI 1.9–5.8, $P < .001$).

TABLE 3.9
Principal component analysis of CISR key area scores (rotated factor matrix)

	Factor 1	Factor 2
Somatic symptoms	0.62	0.1
Fatigue	0.6	0.14
Concentration	0.56	0.2
Sleep complaints	0.57	0.12
Irritability	0.47	0.4
Worry about physical health	0.6	0.06
Depression	0.76	0.07
Depressive ideas	0.73	0.03
Worry	0.63	0.27
Anxiety	0.8	0.17
Phobias	−0.08	0.84
Panic	0.32	0.6

Caseness and positive mental health scores

Four items on positive mental health were randomly distributed in the preliminary SSQ. The presence of any "yea-saying" bias in patient responses to SSQ items was examined by comparing the proportion of cases and noncases who responded to each positive item. Cases were less likely to report positive mental health: (1) feeling happy with life: 29% vs. 62%; OR 0.25, 96% CI 0.1–0.4, $P < .001$; (2) seeing the future with hope: 52% vs. 67%; OR 0.52, 95% CI 0.3–0.8, $P < .01$; (3) thinking clearly: 59% vs. 85%; OR 0.26, 95% CI 0.1–0.4, $P < .001$; and (4) feeling contented: 43% vs. 70%; OR 0.32, 95% CI 0.2–0.5, $P < .001$.

Means of total of positive mental health item scores (range 0–4) were greater for noncases (2.8, SD 1.3 vs. 1.8, SD 1.3; $z = -6.1$, $P < .001$).

Items of the preliminary SSQ which discriminate
cases from noncases

As explained earlier, the 56 items of the preliminary SSQ were reduced to 32 items for further analysis. Discriminant analysis was chosen as the statistical procedure to determine which of the 32 items best predicted mental disorder (with the gold standard of caseness being the outcome). The discriminant analysis was based on forward stepwise selection of items based on Wilks' lambda. Statistically significant discrimination could be achieved with 14 items (see Table 3.10) (canonical $r = 0.64$, lambda $= 0.58$, $\chi^2 (14) = 157.3$, $P < .001$). With this model, 80.7% of noncases and 80% of cases were correctly classified and the overall misclassification rate was 19.3%. Based on these results, the 14-item Shona Symptom Questionnaire was developed (see Fig. 3.1). The total of these 14 items was computed for each patient leading to a final SSQ score which was then used for evaluation of the validity of the SSQ.

Evaluating the psychometric properties of the SSQ

The SSQ was analysed in five ways.

Distribution of scores. T tests were computed to compare the means between cases and noncases for three sets of criteria, viz., gold standard caseness ($n = 100$), etic caseness (CISR scores greater than 12; $n = 156$) and emic caseness (care provider judgment of mental disorder; $n = 179$) (see Table 3.11). SSQ scores were statistically significantly higher for cases on all three criteria.

Validity coefficients. These were computed using the gold standard of caseness as the criterion. A cut-off score of 7–8 for the SSQ provided an

TABLE 3.10
Stepwise discriminant analysis of 32 preliminary SSQ items

Item		Wilks' lambda
1.	Tearfulness	0.79
2.	Poor sleep	0.69
3.	Difficulty enjoying	0.66
4.	Perceptual symptoms	0.64
5.	Suicidal ideas	0.62
6.	Tiredness	0.61
7.	Stomach ache	0.61
8.	Daily work suffering	0.6
9.	Difficulty making decisions	0.6
10.	Thinking too much	0.59
11.	Lack of concentration	0.59
12.	Being startled/panic	0.58
13.	Irritability	0.58
14.	Disturbing dreams	0.58

Two-tailed P values for all items < .001.

optimal balance of sensitivity (71%) and specificity (83%), with a positive predictive value of 66% and negative predictive value of 83%. The area under the ROC curve was computed as 0.88, *SE* 0.02 (Fig. 3.2).

Convergent validity. This was estimated by examining the relationship between SSQ scores and patients' self-assessment of the emotional nature of their illness. Those who felt that their illness was purely somatic ($n = 143$) had lower SSQ scores than those who felt it also involved the mind or soul ($n = 157$): somatic (mean SSQ score 4.4, 95% CI 3.8–4.9) vs. mind/soul (mean 6.7, 95% CI 6.1–7.3; $P < .001$).

Divergent validity. This was estimated by examining the relationship between the SSQ scores and the total score of the four items on positive mental health. The negative correlations between the total positive mental health and SSQ scores were statistically significant ($r = -0.54$, $P < .001$).

TABLE 3.11
Mean SSQ scores for cases and noncases according to different case criteria

Criterion	Case mean (95% CI)	Noncases mean (95% CI)	Two-tailed P
Gold standard case	8.6 (7.9–8.2)	4.1 (3.6–4.5)	< .001
Etic case	7.9 (7.4–8.4)	3.1 (2.6–3.4)	< .001
Emic case	6.2 (5.6–6.8)	4.7 (4.1–5.3)	< .001

Musvondo rapfuura ...
(During the course of the past week ...)

1. ... *pane pamaimboona muchinyanya kufungisisa kana kufunga zvakawanda here?*
   ... did you have times in which you were thinking deep or thinking about many things?
2. ... *pane pamaimbotadza kuisa pfungwa dzenyu pamwechete here?*
   ... did you find yourself at some times failing to concentrate?
3. ... *maimboshatirwa kana kuita hasha zvenhando here?*
   ... did you lose your temper or get annoyed over trivial matters?
4. ... *maimborota hope dzinotyisa kana dzisina kunaka here?*
   ... did you have a nightmare or bad dreams?
5. ... *maimboona kana kunzwa zvinhu zvangazvisingaonekwe kana kunzwikwa nevamwe here?*
   ... did you sometimes see or hear things which others would not see or hear?
6. ... *mudumbu menyu maimborwadza here?*
   ... was your stomach aching?
7. ... *maimbovhundutswa nezvinhu zvisina maturo here?*
   ... were you frightened by trivial things?
8. ... *maimbotadza kurara kana kushaya hope here?*
   ... did you sometimes fail to sleep or lose sleep?
9. ... *pane pamaimbonzwa muchiomerwa neupenyu zvekuti makambochema kana kuti* makambonzwa kuda kuchema here?
   ... were there moments when you felt life was so tough that you cried or wanted to cry?
10. ... *maimbonzwa kuneta here?*
    ... did you feel run down (tired)?
11. ... *pane pamaimboita pfungwa dzekuda kuzviuraya here?*
    ... did you, at times, feel like committing suicide?
12. ... *mainzwa kusafara here mune zvamaiita zuva nezuva?*
    ... did you find it difficult to enjoy your daily activities?
13. ... *basa renyu raive rave kusarira mumashure here?*
    ... was your work lagging behind?
14. ... *mainzwa zvichikuomerai here kuti muzive kuti moita zvipi?*
    ... did you feel you had problems in deciding what to do?

All items are coded either No (score 0) or Yes (Score 1)

FIG. 3.1 The final version of the Shona Symptom Questionnaire

Reliability coefficients. Two statistical measures of internal homogeneity and consistency were computed: Cronbach's alpha = 0.85; and Guttmann's split-half coefficient = 0.84.

RELATIONSHIP BETWEEN BIOMEDICAL AND INDIGENOUS MODELS OF ILLNESS

This section presents data from the SSQ Study.

Emic and etic criteria for caseness

As described earlier, participants in the SSQ study could be classified as cases on either etic, emic, gold standard (agreement between etic and emic) or self-assessment criteria. This section examines the relationship between

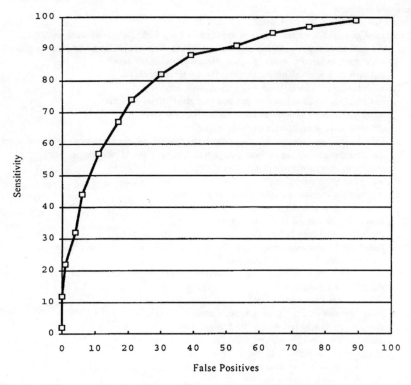

FIG. 3.2 ROC curve plotted for SSQ cut-off scores against gold standard of caseness.

the etic and emic criteria of caseness. For the total sample, agreement between the two sets of criteria was 55% (kappa 0.1). The number of etic cases identified by the care provider (64%) was higher than the number of emic cases identified by CISR (56%). Overall agreement between TMP and etic criteria was 56% (kappa 0.14); 82% of etic cases were identified by the TMP whereas 53% of emic cases were identified by the CISR. Corresponding figures in PHC were: 55% overall agreement (kappa 0.1); 49% of etic cases identified by care provider and 61% of emic cases identified by CISR. Based upon these two criteria, participants could be further grouped into four categories (see Table 3.12): (1) both emic and etic classified as noncase ($n = 67$); (2) emic case/etic noncase ($n = 79$); (3) etic case/emic provider noncase ($n = 56$); and (4) both emic and etic classified as case ($n = 100$)

SSQ scores for the sample categorised into four groups as described above are presented in Table 3.15. A oneway analysis of variance of SSQ scores was statistically significant ($F = 80.1$, $P < .001$). SSQ scores were

TABLE 3.12
Classification of sample according to emic and etic case criteria

Group	Total n = 302 % (n)	TMP n = 150 % (n)	PHC n = 152 % (n)	SSQ score mean 95% CI	Positive mental health score mean 95% CI
1 (Emic and etic noncase)	22 (67)	17 (25)	28 (42)	2.9 2.4–3.5	3.2 2.9–3.4
2 (Emic case, etic noncase)	26 (79)	35 (53)	17 (26)	3.1 2.5–3.7	3.2 3–3.5
3 (Etic case, emic noncase)	18 (56)	9 (13)	28 (43)	6.8 6–7.5	1.9 1.5–2.3
4 (Etic and emic case)	33 (100)	39 (59)	27 (41)	8.6 7.9–9.2	1.8 1.6–2.1

highest for the cases and lowest for noncases; group 2 scores were similar to noncases while group 3 scores were marginally lower than cases. A oneway analysis of variance of positive mental health scores was statistically significant ($F = 32.3$, $P < .001$). Scores for each group are presented in Table 3.12. Noncases had the highest positive mental health scores and cases the lowest. Group 2 had positive mental health scores similar to noncases while group 3 had scores similar to cases.

Another criterion of caseness was the participants' own assessment of the nature of their illness. Half of them felt that their illness had an emotional component (as determined by their response that the illness had affected their mind/soul: $n = 157$, 52%). The level of agreement was highest with the gold standard case criterion (overall 61%; kappa 0.23) followed by the etic criterion (overall 61%; kappa 0.21) and the emic criterion (overall 60%; kappa 0.19).

Kufungisisa (thinking too much) and psychiatric morbidity

The sample was classified on the basis of their answers to the question "do you feel your illness has been caused by kufungisisa?". More than half the patients (62%; $n = 187$) felt that kufungisisa was a probable cause for their illness (Kf patients). Kf patients were older (31.4 years, SD 12 vs. 28.6 years, SD 12.2, $t = 2.01$, $P = .04$). They were more likely to be female (68% vs. 50.5%, OR 2.1, 95% CI 1.3–3.4, $P < .01$), and to be unemployed (66% vs. 49%, OR 2, 95% CI 1.2-3.4, $P < .01$). After adjustment for both these variables, only gender remained statistically significantly associated with the Kf causal model ($P = .04$). There was no difference in chronicity of illness between the two groups. Kf patients were more likely to consider that their illness had affected their mind/soul (73% vs. 27%, OR 11.7, 95% CI 6.6–20.7, $P < .001$) and were more likely to consider supernatural factors as being causally related (57% vs. 39%, OR 2, 95% CI 1.3–3.3, $P < .01$).

Mental illness and Kufungisisa.   The hypothesis was that the indigenous construct of *kufungisisa* was associated with biomedical constructs of CMD. This hypothesis was examined in the following way:

- Phenomenology: The 56 idioms of the preliminary SSQ were compared between Kf and nonKf groups; 40 items were found to be commoner in the Kf group ($P < .05$). A discriminant analysis with forward stepwise selection was carried out with these 40 items of the preliminary SSQ with belief in *kufungisisa* being a causal factor being the outcome. Statistically significant discrimination was Kf achieved with 13 items (canonical $r = 0.58$, Wilks' lambda $= 0.69$, χ^2 (12) $= 107.6$, $P < .001$). Most items were related to the biomedical construct of mixed anxiety–depression (see Table 3.13).
- Severity of morbidity: Two measures of the severity of morbidity were analysed for the two groups, the 14-item SSQ and the Revised

TABLE 3.13

Stepwise discriminant analysis of idioms of distress predicting that patients believe that *kufungisisa* (thinking too much) had caused their illness

Idiom	Wilks' lambda
1. Worrying about life's problems	0.8
2. Thinking too much	0.76
3. Palpitations	0.74
4. Lacking energy/feeling weak	0.72
5. Worrying about one's health	0.73
6. Becoming forgetful	0.72
7. Headache	0.71
8. Difficulty making decisions	0.71
9. Lacking concentration	0.7
10. Feeling that one's behaviour had changed	0.7
11. Tiredness	0.69
12. Not feeling like speaking or being spoken to	0.69
13. Pains in the side	0.69

Two-tailed P values for all variables $< .001$.

TABLE 3.14

Comparison of morbidity scores and case classification between patients who believe that *kufungisisa* did or did not cause their illness

Morbidity scores

Measure (range of scores)	Kufungisisa mean (SD) 95% CI	*Not* Kufungisisa mean (SD) 95% CI	Mann–Whitney, two-tailed P
SSQ	6.5 (3.6)	4 (3.5)	z = −5.8
(0–14)	6–7	3.3-4.6	< .001
CISR	15.6 (10.7)	9.3 (8.4)	z = −4.9
(0–57)	14–17	7.8–10.9	< .001

Case classification

Criterion	Kf case %	Non Kf case %	OR, 95% CI	P value
Etic	61.5	36	2.9, 1.8–4.7	< .001
Emic	71	56.5	1.9, 1.1–3.1	< .01
Gold standard	74	56	2.2, 1.3–3.8	< .001
Patient self-assessment	87	12	11.7, 6.6–20.7	< .001

Clinical Interview Schedule. Scores were higher for the Kf group for both measures (see Table 3.14).

- Classification as cases: Kf patients were more likely to be classified as cases on all four criteria of case classification, in particular patient self-assessment (Table 3.14).

Supernatural causation and psychiatric morbidity

The open question "What do you call your illness" probed the nature of the causal model for the illness. About 10% of the sample ($n = 30$) mentioned a supernatural label. The commonest label used was *chivanhu* ($n = 15$), literally meaning an illness of the people, referring to the indigenous African people. This term implies illness caused through supernatural causes, in particular witchcraft. In two instances, the patient elaborated that the illness had been caused by the *mudzimu* (ancestral spirits) wanting to "come out". The remaining patients felt their illness was the result of witchcraft and some mentioned *mamhepo* (bad airs/evil spirits) and *zvishiri* (birds used in witchcraft) as specific types of bewitchment.

The definition of supernatural causation was based on the responses of patients to the closed question "Do you feel that factors such as witchcraft may have caused your illness?"; half the sample responded positively and were classified as the supernatural group (S; $n = 151$) and the rest were classified in the nonsupernatural group (NS; $n = 151$).

Comparing supernatural and nonsupernatural groups. Supernatural patients were more likely to present with psychological complaints (e.g."thinking too much"), relationship problems (e.g. "my husband has a girlfriend"), and social problems (e.g. unemployment) (15% vs. 3%, $\chi^2 = 10.4$, $P < .001$). There was no difference in age or gender between the two groups. Subjects in the supernatural group were more likely to have been TMP attenders; to be unemployed; not to have completed school; to have a chronic illness; to perceive that their illness involved their mind/soul; and to consider that *kufungisisa* had caused their illness (see Table 3.15). After adjustment for all variables in Table 3.15 and age and gender, all variables other than unemployment remained associated ($P < .05$) with supernatural models of causation.

Mental disorder and supernatural causation. The relationship between the model of supernatural causation and mental disorder hypothesis was examined in the following manner.

- Phenomenology: The 56 idioms of the preliminary SSQ were compared between S and NS groups; 13 items were found to be commoner in the S group ($P < .05$). These 13 items were entered into a forward stepwise discriminant analysis to determine which items best predicted membership of the supernatural group. Six items were extracted (canonical correlation = 0.29, Wilks' lambda = 0.91, χ^2

TABLE 3.15
Comparison of sociodemographic and explanatory model variables between participants who did or did not believe that supernatural factors caused their illness

Variable	Proportion of S group (%)	Proportion of NS group (%)	OR; 95% CI two-tailed P
Attender site:			
TMP attenders	73	26	7.4; 4.5–12.4 < .001
Chronicity:			
Illness > 1 month	71	32	5.2; 3.2–8.5 < .001
Employment:			
Unemployed	80	67	1.9; 1.1–3.3 < .05
Education:			
not completed school	82	71	1.9; 1.1–3.2 < .05
Emotional origins of illness:			
Illness involved the mind/soul	66	38	2.9; 1.9–4.8 < .001
Kufungisisa caused the illness	70	54	2; 1.3–3.3 < .01

TABLE 3.16
Stepwise discriminant analysis of idioms of distress predicting that patients believed
that supernatural factors had caused their illness

Item	Wilks' lambda
Feeling tense, nervous, or anxious	0.96
Worrying about life's problems	0.94
Abdominal discomfort after meals/feeling bloated	0.93
Sensation of things moving around/within the body	0.92
Trouble thinking clearly	0.91
Feeling as if one was losing one's senses	0.91

Two-tailed P values for all variables $< .001$.

(6) = 27.76, $P < .001$). All six items are conceptually related to the biomedical construct of anxiety (see Table 3.16).

- Severity of morbidity: Two measures of the severity of morbidity were analysed for the two groups, the SSQ and the CISR. Scores were higher for the S group for both measures, the difference being statistically significant for the SSQ (see Table 3.17).
- Classification as cases: Supernatural participants were more likely to be classified as cases on three of the four criteria (see Table 3.17).

TABLE 3.17
Comparison of morbidity scores and case classification between patients who did or
did not believe that supernatural factors had caused their illness

Morbidity scores

Measure (range of scores)	Supernatural mean (SD) 95% CI	Nonsupernatural mean (SD) 95% CI	Mann–Whitney, two-tailed P
SSQ	6.2 (3.8)	5 (3.6)	$z = -2.5$
(0–14)	5.5–6.7	4.4–5.6	< .01
CISR	14.2 (10.5)	12.3 (10.1)	$z = -1.4$
(0–57)	12.4–15.8	10.6–13.9	.1

Case classification

Criterion	Sp case %	Nonsp case %	OR, 95% CI	P value
Etic	54.5	45	1.4, 0.9–2.3	.1
Emic	66	40	2.9, 1.8–5.5	< .001
Gold standard	60	45	1.8, 1.1–2.9	< .01
Patient self-assessment	63	36	2.9, 1.9–4.8	< .001

PREVALENCE, ASSOCIATIONS, AND RISK FACTORS OF CMD

The data on prevalence were derived from the SSQ Study as a result of its cross-sectional study design while data on associations and risk factors are from the Case–Control Study.

The prevalence of psychiatric morbidity in PHC and TMP attenders

This was examined according to four case criteria: emic, etic, the gold standard of caseness, and patient self-assessment of the emotional nature of their illness. Except for etic criteria, the prevalence of psychiatric morbidity was higher in TMP attenders, being statistically significant for the emic case, the gold standard of caseness, and the patient self-assessment criteria (see Table 3.18). After adjustment for age and gender, the association of being a TMP attender and caseness remained statistically significant for the emic (OR 3.5, 95% CI 2.1–5.8, $P < .001$), the gold standard (OR 1.6, 95% CI 1.02–2.7, $P < .05$) and the patient self-assessment criteria (OR 2.3, 95% CI 1.4–3.8, $P < .001$).

The associations and risk factors of CMD

Of the participants initially approached after sampling and who satisfied eligibility criteria, 17 did not give consent for the Case–Control Study of which 11 were from GP surgeries. A total of 396 subjects were recruited, of whom 199 were likely cases (C) and 197 were likely noncases (NC) based on their SSQ scores. PHC attenders accounted for 36% of the sample (C = 72; NC = 71), GP attenders 31% (C = 60; NC = 62) and TMP attenders 33% (C = 67; NC = 64).

GP, PHC and TMP attenders in either group did not differ from one another on the following variables: age, sex, number of children, accommodation status, BDQ scores at recruitment, and number of presenting complaints. PHC and TMP cases had higher SSQ scores than

TABLE 3.18
Prevalence of psychiatric morbidity according to four case criteria

Case criterion	TMP preval. %	PHC preval. %	OR 95% CI	Two-tailed P
Etic	48	55	0.7 0.5–1.2	.1
Emic	75	44	3.7 2.2–6.3	< .001
Gold standard	39	27	1.7 1.1–2.8	< .05
Patient self-assessment	64	40	2.6 1.6–4.1	< .001

GP cases (mean 9.7, *SD* 1.5 vs. 9.2, *SD* 1.3; $t = 2.3$, $P = .02$) and had fewer years of formal education ($P < .001$). PHC and TMP participants in both groups had lower incomes than GP participants ($P < .001$). TMP participants in both groups were more likely to be unemployed ($P < .001$) and to have an illness longer than one month ($P < .001$). Due to these differences, all adjustments for associations with caseness included site of recruitment (in addition to age and sex).

Sociodemographic data. Cases were more likely to be women (see Table 3.19); to be older (mean 34.5 years, *SD* 12.8 vs. 31.8, *SD* 11.2; $t = 2.2$, $P = .02$); and to have fewer years of formal education (mean 7.8, *SD* 3.5 vs. 9, *SD* 3.3; $t = 3.4$, $P < .001$) than noncases. Associations with unemployment and not having passed O levels in school, were not statistically significant after adjustment for age and sex (see Table 3.19).

Economic variables. A total of 63% of cases and 57% of noncases lived in their own home with an average of 2–3 rooms and 4–5 members in the household, as defined in the Zimbabwe census as all persons living in the same house who share meals (Central Statistical Office, 1995). Household income data was volunteered by 216 participants who were

TABLE 3.19
Associations of sociodemographic and economic variables with CMD

Variable	Direction of association % cases vs. % noncases	Simple OR (95% CI) P values	Adjusted OR (95% CI) P values
Gender	Female 65% vs. 55%	1.45 (0.97–2.17) .04	1.5 (1.01–2.29)[1] .04
Age	Continuous Cases older	1.01 (1–1.03) .02	1.02 (1–1.03)[2] .01
Educational qualification	O levels not passed 67% vs. 57%	1.5 (0.99–2.2) .05	1.17 (0.7–1.8) .46
Occupation	Unemployed 46% vs. 35.5%	1.5 (1–2.3) .03	1.5 (0.96–2.3) .07
Being unable to buy food due to lack of money in previous month	44% vs. 26%	2.2 (1.4-3.4) < .0001	2.1 (1.4–3.3) < .0001
Cash savings	38% vs. 59%	.43 (0.28–0.64) < .0001	.45 (0.3–0.68) < .0001
Covered by medical aid	24% vs. 34.5%	.58 (0.37–0.91) .01	.6 (0.38–0.93) .02

[1] Adjusted for age and site.
[2] Adjusted for sex and site.

employed; the mean monthly income was less in cases (Zim$673, *SD* 596 vs. Zim$991, *SD* 972; $z = -2.6$, $P = .008$).

Just over a third of the sample reported being in debt (35%). When reasons for being in debt were analysed, a greater proportion of cases in debt reported costs incurred in consultations, medication, or lost income due to their illness as compared to noncases in debt (25% vs. 8%, $\chi^2 = 17.8$, $P < .001$). A greater proportion of cases perceived their debt as being moderately or severely stressful (50% vs. 26%; $\chi^2 = 8.6$, $P = .003$). Cases were more likely to have been unable to buy food due to lack of money in the previous month, and were less likely to have cash savings, or to be covered by a medical aid insurance scheme (Table 3.19). After adjustment for all three variables, the associations of being unable to buy food (OR 1.7, 95% CI 1.1–2.7, $P < .01$) and having cash savings (OR 0.5, 95% CI 0.35–0.8, $P < .01$) remained statistically significant.

Clinical and explanatory model data. Somatic symptoms were the commonest presenting symptoms in cases and noncases. The combination of one or more of four pains (stomach, head, chest/heart, back) were commoner in cases (48% vs. 33%, OR 1.9, 95% CI 1.1–4.5, $P = .002$). Alcohol use as measured by the AUDIT was not associated with caseness. Cases were more likely to have an illness longer than one month; to have three or more presenting complaints; to have a psychosocial causal model of their illness; to believe that witchcraft and *kufungisisa* had caused their illness; to feel that their illness had an emotional component; and to have a history of "stress" or psychiatric problems in the past (Table 3.20). Qualitative data on the stress revealed a range of themes with sickness or death in the immediate family, poverty and its implications on feeding one's family or educating children, and marital conflict being the commonest. After adjusting for all variables in Table 3.20 (and sex, age, and site), statistically significant associations with caseness were found for (1) more than three presenting complaints (OR 2, 95% CI 1.2–3.5, $P < .01$); (2) belief in witchcraft as a causal agent (OR 2.2, 95% CI 1.1–4.5, $P < .05$); (3) belief in *kufungisisa* as causal agent (OR 2.6, 95% CI 1.3–5.3, $P < .01$).

Family, social, and personal variables. Associations of caseness with loss of mother, loss of both parents, lack of a rural home and four or more children (for female cases) were not statistically significant after adjustment (Table 3.21).

Life events. Whilst cases had a tendency to experience stressful life events in the previous 12 months more frequently, statistically significant differences were found for only a handful of events and difficulties, viz.

TABLE 3.20
Association of clinical variables and explanatory models with CMD

Variable	Direction of association % cases vs. % noncases	Simple OR (95% CI) P values	Adjusted OR (95% CI) P values
Length of illness	>1 month	2.2 (1.5–3.3)	2.3 (1.5–3.7)
	55% vs. 35%	<.0001	<.0001
Number of presenting complaints	3 or more	2.3 (1.5–3.4)	2.2 (1.4–3.3)
	51% vs. 31%	<.0001	<.0001
Causal explanatory model	Psychosocial	1.7 (1.13–2.8)	1.8 (1.1–2.9)
	46% vs. 32%	.01	.01
Witchcraft $n = 329$	Belief as causal	2.3 (1.4–3.9)	2.76 (1.6–4.8)
	29% vs. 15%	.001	<.0001
Kufungisisa $n = 383$	Belief as causal	4.2 (2.7–6.5)	4.1 (2.6–6.2)
	66% vs. 31%	<.0001	<.0001
Mind-somatic origin of illness	Mind is involved	2.8 (1.8–4.2)	2.7 (1.7–4.1)
	61% vs. 36%	<.0001	<.0001
History of "stress"	Positive	2.3 (1.5–3.5)	2.2 (1.4–3.4)
	72% vs. 52%	<.0001	<.0001

loss of job (14.5% vs. 10%; adjusted OR 2; 95% CI 1.05–3.8, $P = .03$) and the experience of infertility (8.5% vs. 2%, adjusted OR 4.9; 95% CI 1.6–15.2, $P = .005$). Sickness in a family relative was associated with caseness, but had an opposite effect for the two sexes; male cases were more likely to have experienced this (adjusted OR 2.2, 95% CI 1.05–4.4, $P = .03$) while female cases were less likely (adjusted OR 0.53, 95% CI 0.3–0.9, $P = .03$). Probing on the emotional response to the event revealed that although cases tended to perceive events as being more stressful, this was not statistically significant.

Disability. The ability to work (including being absent from formal employment, household duties, peasant farming, the ability to look for a job) was more likely to be impaired in cases (62% vs. 41%, OR 2.3, 95% CI 1.5–3.5, $P < .001$). Greater numbers of noncases reported no disruption of their daily lives (23% vs. 11%, OR 2.3, 95% CI 1.3–4.1, $P = .002$). Total scores on the BDQ were higher for cases (mean 8.3, SD 5.6 vs. 6.5, SD 5.3; $z = -3.2$, $P = .001$). Cases spent twice the number of days in the previous month being unable to work (mean 6, SD 9 vs. 3.3, SD 6; $z = -3.6$, $P = .001$) and twice the number of days bedridden (mean 2.9, SD 5.5 vs. 1.5, SD 4.3; $z = -4.5$, $P < .001$). The subjective perception of overall quality of life was worse for cases with 39% rating this as being unsatisfactory as compared to 26% of noncases (adjusted OR 1.9, 95% CI 1.2–2.9, $P = .004$).

TABLE 3.21
Associations of family, social and personal variables with CMD

Variable	Direction of association % cases vs. % noncases	Simple OR (95% CI) P values	Adjusted OR (95% CI) P values
Mother dead	32.5% vs. 21%	1.8 (1.1–2.8) .01	1.5 (0.9–2.5) .09
Both parents dead	26.5% vs. 15%	1.9 (1.2–3.2) .007	1.6 (0.9–3) .09
No rural home	89% vs. 94%	0.5 (0.2–1.06) .07	0.5 (0.2–1.17) .12
Number of children (for women only, $n=235$)	4 or more 38% vs. 25%	1.8 (1.03–3.2) 0.03	1.48 (0.7–3.1)[1] 0.29

[1] Adjusted for site and age only.

Pathways to care.   The first care provider consulted for the current problem was a biomedical provider for about 80% of both groups and a TMP for the remainder. In the previous year, cases were more likely to have consulted a PHC (66% vs. 58%; adjusted OR 1.5, 95% CI 0.99–2.2, $P=.05$); a TMP (60% vs. 44%; adjusted OR 2.3, 5% CI 1.4–3.7, $P=.001$); and to have sought advice from a formal church-based pastor or priest (17% vs. 9%; adjusted OR 2, 95% CI 1.1–3.8, $P=.02$). Although cases showed a trend to have a greater number of consultations with all care providers in the previous month, these were not statistically significant.

Care provider diagnosis and treatment.   PHC and GP attenders: Care provider assessment data was available for 252 of the 265 attenders. When asked to state the primary diagnosis, nurses and GPs were more likely to choose a psychological disorder for cases (20% vs. 9%; OR 2.6, 95% CI 1.1–5.9, $P=.01$). The commonest somatic diagnoses were: acute respiratory tract infections (13–15%); sexually transmitted diseases and urinary tract infections (11%); gastritis, dyspepsia, and diarrheal disease (10%); and skin and eye infections (10–15%). No differences were found in rates of any specific physical illnesses diagnosed. HIV status was never recorded due to reasons of confidentiality; diagnoses given were usually those of AIDS-related diseases such as pneumonia. Infertility was diagnosed in just one patient. Although cases were more likely to be prescribed parenteral (32% vs. 26%) or oral medication (91% vs. 85%), these differences were not statistically significant. The commonest parenteral medication was penicillin, and the commonest oral medications were analgesics, antibiotics, and antacids. Psychotropics were more frequently prescribed for cases (9% vs. 4%); these were most often benzodiazepines.

TMP attenders: TMP assessment data was collected for all 131 attenders. TMP were more likely to consider that the illness in cases had been caused by witchcraft (52% vs. 36%; adjusted OR 2.3, 95% CI 1.1–4.7, $P = .02$) or by *kufungisisa* (66% vs. 45%; adjusted OR 2.6, 95% CI 1.3–5.2, $P = .009$).

CHAPTER FOUR

Discussion

LIMITATIONS OF THE RESEARCH
METHODOLOGY

Ethnographic Study

A limitation was the obvious gender bias in the composition of the care providers in the study sample. However, it is widely acknowledged that women are overrepresented in certain carer groups such as nurses, VHWs, and those caring for sick relatives in the home. Focus group discussions were used as a qualitative research method because they can facilitate the eliciting of views from a relatively large number of care providers while being time and cost effective; however, the limitations of FGD as compared to qualitative interviews and participant observation are recognised (Khan & Manderson, 1992). Thus, data collected through FGD may be influenced by biases operating in a group such as peer pressure by other participants. The focus group is best characterised as a complementary tool which supports data gathered by other research methods; in the Ethnographic Study, FGD were used to elicit data on concepts of mental illness which were to be evaluated in subsequent stages. Further, there was already a body of ethnographic data on mental illness in Zimbabwe (Gelfand, 1967) and the FGD did not aim to be an exhaustive account of indigenous models of illness.

Phenomenology Study

A potential limitation of this study is that patients were not selected on a random basis; thus consecutive attenders were recruited on the grounds that the care provider suspected a psychological illness or because the patient fitted the screening criteria given to the care provider as a guideline. However, the aim of this study was exploratory and the symptoms generated were to be subjected to further analysis in the SSQ Study. Indeed, by selecting patients with conspicuous psychiatric morbidity as identified by TMPs and primary care nurses, this study was following the principles of the "new" cross-cultural psychiatry. Another limitation was the essentially static concept of explanatory models which was inherent in a cross-sectional study. The author recognises that, in reality, "illness explanations are dynamic entities that fluctuate with time in ways that allow them to be meaningfully incorporated into the mesh of ongoing life circumstances" (Hunt, Jordan, & Irwin, 1989). However, the aim of this study was not to examine the nature of this process or its relationship to ongoing life circumstances.

SSQ and Case–Control Studies

A number of limitations are recognised in the SSQ and Case–Control Studies. One source of bias could have resulted from the selection of only those TMPs who saw at least five patients a day. This may have biased the figures on agreement between emic and etic case criteria since it could be possible that those TMPs who had higher numbers of attenders were more likely to be informed of biomedical concepts. The sampling frame of TMPs had been defined by a community survey in the two study suburbs; in this survey, nearly a third reported that they only saw patients at weekends. The majority of TMPs stated that they were consulted, on average, by two to three patients a day (Winston et al., 1995). If a random sample of TMPs had been selected from this sampling frame, it would have been likely that the recruitment would have taken much longer and may not have been logistically feasible. Thus, a smaller sampling frame of only those TMPs who saw at least five patients a day was created and TMP were selected for the study randomly from this frame.

A site-related bias may have been likely at PHC in connection with items relating to supernatural causation of illness. It was possible that PHC subjects may have been less forthcoming about such beliefs due to the risk of appearing "primitive". Attempts were made to reduce this bias by giving a general statement to the effect that "many people in Zimbabwe feel that their illness is related to supernatural factors." It was felt that this would, at the very least, reassure the participant that the interviewers were open to the possibility that the participant believed that supernatural factors had caused their illness and that no value judgment would be made. Further, it was stressed at the start of the interview that the information collected was strictly confidential and would not be shared with the PHC staff (since some nursing staff were sceptical about the use of traditional medicine).

Two limitations were acknowledged during the selection of the emic criterion of caseness. First, there was the problem of the lack of standardisation. Thus, concepts of mental illness can vary considerably between different health care providers being influenced by a number of factors such as their views of illness causation, length of experience, specific experience in mental health, age, and religion. For example, nurses with mental health training may have been more likely to identify cases of CMD along biomedical lines as compared to their counterparts, while *n'anga* may have had different diagnostic concepts to *profita* because of the latter's belief in Christianity. This lack of standardisation was the main reason for not using the emic criterion as the gold standard of caseness. Instead, agreement between the emic criterion and the criterion of caseness based on a standardised (and field-tested) psychiatric interview was used as the gold standard. The second potential limitation was the use of the judgment of general nurses as an emic criterion of caseness. It is possible that using nurses' judgment may have inflated the agreement levels between emic and etic criteria. It can be argued that biomedical health workers, by virtue of having been trained in what is historically a Euro-American system of medicine, may not be regarded as holding emic views about illness. According to this view, only TMPs can be considered to have a truly emic view. However, the experience of the author suggested otherwise. General nurses form the frontline of primary health care in Zimbabwe. The psychiatric component of the training emphasises psychotic disorders, epilepsy, and organic mental disorders as per the recommended priorities for low-income countries (Essex & Gosling, 1983). All the nurses were indigenous Zimbabweans who had trained in Zimbabwe and lived their working lives in the high-density suburbs of Harare. Furthermore, emic views are not synonymous with traditional views; thus, cultures are dynamic entities with certain values and ideas giving way to others or coexisting with new alternatives. Thus, the diagnostic opinion of general nurses reflected the combined clinical and personal life experiences of these health care professionals in the Zimbabwean environment and were considered as an emic judgment.

The studies did not lead to the generation of specific psychiatric diagnostic categories as per ICD-10 classification. However, the categorical classification of CMD is fraught with conceptual and clinical problems and may lack validity in primary care populations (Patel, 1996; Tyrer, 1996). Thus, it was considered more useful to present data on psychiatric symptoms according to the symptom groups represented in the key areas of the Revised Clinical Interview Schedule. The relationship between the key areas were further analysed by principal component analysis, the findings of which suggested that most symptom groups of CMD were highly related to one another and only panic and phobias loaded on a different factor. This issue is discussed later.

There may be a circularity in estimating psychometric properties of the SSQ from the same data set which led to its development. However, the main psychometric properties of validity were evaluated against independent criteria, e.g. patients' perception of illness causation and items on positive mental health, and were thus unlikely to be exaggerated. Sensitivity of the scale to change, its usefulness in different clinical populations and reliability measures such as interrater reliability and test–retest reliability were not estimated due to the fact that the SSQ was the outcome of the SSQ Study. Some of the psychometric properties of the SSQ have been evaluated in subsequent studies which have shown that the SSQ scores are sensitive to change against the criterion of patient perception of overall health (Patel et al., 1997d).

PRESENTATION AND ASSESSMENT OF CMD

Somatisation and common mental disorder

Somatisation is the process which involves the presentation of somatic complaints for a psychological illness wherein the patient does not acknowledge the non-somatic origins of their distress (Bridges & Goldberg, 1985). Low recognition of CMD by health workers has been partly attributed to this process. Somatisation has been typically stated to be more common in low-income countries and in ethnic minorities in developed societies. This concept has been challenged by other authors on the grounds that many somatic presentations may represent real somatic sensations arising from psychological morbidity (such as tension headaches) and somatic metaphors which are conceptually used to communicate psychological distress (Mumford, 1993). Further, there is evidence that somatic presentations are common in Euro-American societies as well. Indeed, some authors argue that "from the cross-cultural perspective, it is not somatisation but psychologization in the West that appears unusual and requires explanation" (Kleinman & Kleinman, 1985).

Although somatic complaints were the commonest reasons for consultation in the phenomenology, SSQ and Case–Control Studies, patients with a CMD freely admitted to the cognitive symptoms which predominate in the final version of the SSQ (see below) and were more likely to attribute their illness to an emotional problem. Thus somatic presentations were often superficial presentations of a process of the clinical evaluation of personal distress. These findings are consistent with Dhadphale, Cooper, and Cartwright-Taylor (1989), whose cross-sectional survey in Kenyan district hospitals showed that "although somatic symptoms dominate the clinical presentation, a health worker can invariably find evidence of psychological or emotional phenomena." Similar findings have been reported from other low-income societies (Araya, Robert, Richard, & Lewis, 1994; Channabasavanna et al., 1993). These findings contradict the popular beliefs regarding the high frequency of somatisation in low-income countries. At least part of this contradictory finding may be accounted for by the way the question on perceived origin or attribution of illness is asked. As described earlier, in many African cultures the concept of the mind included the heart, soul, or spirit centres and illnesses may be perceived as arising from any of these sources. If the concept of the spirit, soul, or social problems were included in the question, many patients admit that their problem was not somatic. Thus, it appears as if somatisation does not occur as an alternative to expressions of emotional distress but as an accompaniment (Kirmayer, 1989).

Rather than being a phenomenon which was earlier considered to be an obstacle to the successful management of psychological disorder in primary care, some authors have suggested that somatisation may serve an adaptive role in helping a person avoid introspection and self-blame for failures and disappointments in life and may even prevent persons from becoming severely depressed by protecting them from painful and distressing emotions and cognitions (Bridges, Goldberg, Evans, & Sharpe, 1991; Chaturvedi, 1993). Thus, somatisation may be a form of defence mechanism whereby psychological distress is channelled into somatic complaints thereby preventing a full-fledged nervous breakdown (Ebigbo, Janakiramaiah, & Kumaraswamy, 1989). This model of explaining somatic presentations poses a challenge to the rationale behind the notion that the treatment of CMD with somatisation should be to facilitate the "reattribution" of the illness model to an inner, psychological realm.

Psychiatric phenomenology

Etic phenomenology was elicited using the Revised Clinical Interview Schedule (CISR) in the Phenomenology and SSQ Studies. Three-quarters of the patients with conspicuous psychiatric morbidity in the former study were classified as etic cases on the basis of the cut-off score of 11–12. Most psychological constructs such as depression and anxiety were recorded for the majority of cases. Phobias were never recorded, and obsessions and compulsions were very rare. The non-reporting of phobias was puzzling.

The existence of phobic symptoms in the community had been confirmed in the Ethnographic Study. Back translation of the phobia key question by four independent health professionals showed that the Shona version was linguistically equivalent to the original English text. Thus, it was possible that phobias were either not considered to be a mental illness by primary care providers (and therefore, such patients were not selected for the study) or that phobic patients did not consult primary care providers. The high intraclass coefficient suggested that mental illness constructs were strongly related to each other; one of the highest correlations was between anxiety and depression supporting the dimensional model of CMD (Goldberg & Huxley, 1992).

The SSQ Study CISR data replicated many of the above findings. Anxiety and depression, the commonest key areas of the CISR, were reported by over 90% of cases. In contrast, obsessions or compulsions were rarely reported which is consistent with other work from Africa suggesting that these symptoms are very uncommon (Bertschy & Ahyi, 1991). Principal component analysis of 12 key area scores (excluding obsessions and compulsions) extracted two factors; all but two key areas loaded maximally on the first factor which could be described as a "mixed anxiety–depression" factor. Phobias and panic loaded on the second factor. This analysis suggests that symptom groups of CMD are related to one another along two dimensions: anxiety–depression and panic–phobias. This accords with anecdotal clinical evidence that patients in primary care either tend to have clear-cut panic disorder or a general spectrum of anxiety and depressive symptoms.

The conceptual and clinical validity of the distinction between anxiety and depression in primary care settings is in doubt due to the growing evidence gathered from a variety of sources and the findings of the studies described in this book. Thus, as with many non-Indoeuropean languages, there are no conceptually equivalent terms for anxiety or depression in the Shona language (Chaturvedi, 1993; Ihezue, 1989; Leff, 1977; Manson et al., 1985; Swartz et al., 1985); attempts to find conceptual equivalents often lead to somatic metaphors (such as the "heart is weak" or the "painful heart"; Abas et al., 1994). Factor analyses of CMD from studies from Euro-American and low-income societies often lead to single-factor solutions with anxiety and depression loading on the same factor (Jacob et al., 1997; Lewis, 1992; Ndetei, 1987). Psychiatrists tend to show a perceptual and inferential bias towards rating a distinction between anxiety and depression more so than is actually reported by patients (Lewis, 1991). There is a high degree of comorbidity in studies where the categorical approach is used, notably the WHO multinational studies (Ustun, Simon, & Sartorius, 1995a). But perhaps the most important evidence of the lack of validity of the categorical approach to CMD is that few primary health workers recognise these categories in their patients. Rather than their lack of awareness, in the view of the author, there is sufficient evidence to suggest that anxiety and depression in primary care attenders are probably different symptoms of the same distress syndrome. Thus, in primary care in Harare, a model which includes both anxiety and depression in the same overall clinical category is likely to be a more useful way of conceptualising CMD, although factor analysis and clinical experience suggests that panic disorder may represent a distinct syndrome.

The prevalence of phobic symptoms was higher in the SSQ Study, suggesting that the low prevalence in the Phenomenology Study was probably due to the selection bias of the care providers in the detection of psychiatric morbidity. Despite the higher reporting of such symptoms, however, the actual scores which represent severity of symptomatology were not high. It would appear that clinically significant phobic states are uncommon, a finding consistent with the rare reporting of phobic disorders in Africa (Morakinyo, 1985; Otakpor, 1987). Some authors have argued that the low reporting of phobias is due to the prominence of somatic symptoms and the lack of recognition that phobic stimuli may be unique in the African setting and may not reflect common phobic stimuli in Euro-American cultures (Morakinyo, 1985, 1989). It was of interest to note that disassociative disorders, in the form of conversion symptoms, were not recorded in the study. This could partly be a methodological artifact resulting from the lack of items on disassociative disorder in the CISR. However, a more likely reason is that these disorders character-istically have florid presentations in low-income societies with manic and psychotic features and neurological impairment which lead to the exclusion of such patients from the study or to them bypassing primary care facilities altogether.

Items of the Shona Symptom Questionnaire

Idioms of distress were elicited by open-ended probing of symptoms in the Phenomenology Study. While many symptoms seemed to have obvious etic equivalents, such as tiredness, others were unique to the setting of this study. Some of these unique symptoms such as feelings of heat, moving pains, prickling of the heart, and abdominal discomfort after meals have been associated with neurotic disorders in other African studies (Awaritefe, 1988; Ayorinde, 1977; Ihezue, 1989; Onyemelukwe, Ahmed, & Onyewotu, 1987). The Phenomenology Study and subsequent piloting led to a list of 45 emic phenomena. The version of the preliminary SSQ used in the SSQ Study included these 45 items plus items from the WHO SRQ instrument which had been the only case finding instrument used previously in Zimbabwe. The rationale for adding the SRQ items was that there was a considerable body of experience with the SRQ across Africa which suggested its usefulness. The SSQ study would evaluate which items best predicted mental disorder and, in keeping with the theory of the "new" cross-cultural psychiatry, the final list could be expected to be a combination of etic and emic items. Four items tapping positive aspects of mental health were randomly distributed amongst the items of the preliminary SSQ. All four showed a negative association with caseness thus suggesting that a "yea-saying" bias was not operating. The final version of the SSQ was developed using discriminant analyses to determine which of the preliminary SSQ items predicted caseness.

The SSQ is a 14-item instrument designed to record the presence of 14 symptoms of CMD over the previous seven days (Patel et al., 1997b). The sum of the 14 items (SSQ score, computed by adding all positive responses giving a range of 0–14) was generated for each patient. The SSQ has seven emic items (i.e. derived from those items unique to the preliminary SSQ), four common items (i.e. items common to the preliminary SSQ and SRQ) and three pure SRQ items. It is apparent that even the emic items have satisfactory equivalents in psychiatric phenomenology, a finding consistent with Beiser and Fleming's (1986) reports with Southeast Asian refugees. Just two items are somatic (tiredness and stomach ache) which suggest that although somatic symptoms may be the commonest presentations of CMD, it is the cognitive and behavioural symptoms which have the greatest diagnostic sensitivity. It is possible that some somatic symptoms typically associated with neurotic illness in Euro-American cultures may not have the same diagnostic specificity in this setting due to the relatively greater prevalence of chronic medical conditions which present with similar symptoms. For example, the item on "loss of appetite" may reflect neurotic symptoms in a society where chronic infectious diseases are rare but is unlikely to be as specific in settings where such diseases are common.

A surprising finding was that perceptual symptoms, viz. hallucinatory phenomena, were found to occur in the context of nonpsychotic mental illness. Since such phenomena are more typically associated with psychotic disorders, the cases which admitted to these symptoms were examined more closely. Altogether 20 participants in the SSQ Study reported this symptom, of whom 17 were classified as cases. Most of the patients presented with chest pains, headache, and stomach ache. Analysis of the clinical data revealed that only two patients had a possible psychotic illness, of whom one was not classified as a case due to low CISR scores (a finding in keeping with the purpose of the CISR). These symptoms were commoner in TMP cases (9% vs. 4%, $\chi^2 = 3.5$, $P = .05$). An analysis of the explanatory models and psychiatric symptoms suggested a culture-specific context of these hallucinatory experiences. Thus, many sufferers had high levels of anxiety and believed that supernatural factors, in particular witchcraft, had caused their illness. Their anxiety led to poor sleep and vivid nightmares, often causing them to wake at night. The hallucinations were mostly visual and included objects used in witchcraft, such as owls and *tokoloshi* (small men). It was not clear from this study whether the phenomena could be classifed as pseudo-hallucinations, such as those described in the neurotic condition "*ode ori*" in Nigeria, where symptoms include auditory perceptions such as boiling, hissing, and humming noises which are perceived as arising inside the ears (Makanjuola, 1987). The possibility of the visual phenomena being pseudo-hallucinations is raised by the association of nightmares with CMD in this and other African studies (Awaritefe, 1988; Onyemelukwe ct al., 1987).

Many non-European societies make no distinction between hallucinations and visual imagery associated with culturally sanctioned experiences (Murphy, 1976). Hallucinatory experiences are often attributed to supernatural causes, such as having offended ancestral spirits or being the victim of witchcraft or as an experience indicating that the person will become a shaman. Al-Issa (1995) theorises that the differing meaning of hallucinations is related to the varying degrees of rationality and the distinction between reality and imagination in different societies. In less rational cultures, such as those in Africa, the distinction between reality and imagination is more flexible; individuals may be more likely to experience hallucinations in a wider range of social settings and be more likely to value positively and share their experiences with others. Awareness of the culturally varying significance of hallucinations and increased emphasis on the quality of the experience, e.g. its intrusiveness and persistence, may help in clarifying their diagnostic significance.

Psychometric properties of the SSQ

The Shona Symptom Questionnaire emphasises the number of symptoms versus their severity, creating the risk that a patient with a number of minor symptoms causing little distress may be regarded as a case while those with a few intense symptoms are not (Williams et al., 1980). However, previous experience with the SRQ in Africa had shown that the dichotomous no/yes response format was simple and easy to use in primary care and thus the advantage of simplicity overruled the potential of finer discriminations which ordinal rating codes could provide.

Psychometric properties of the SSQ were evaluated by examining the relationship of the total scores of the 14 items with a number of criteria. Total scores were higher for cases for all three sets of case criteria: etic, emic, and the gold standard. The validity of the SSQ was judged both against the patients' perceptions of the emotional nature of their illness and with items tapping positive aspects of mental health derived from an independent interview on quality of life. In both instances, the instrument performed well, providing evidence of its convergent and divergent validity respectively. Its internal consistency was high, suggesting that the instrument was tapping a relatively homogenous dimension of distress. The area under a ROC (relative operating characteristic) curve is a useful procedure for estimating the discriminating power of a screening instrument. The ROC area under the curve of 0.88 for the SSQ is high and is comparable to screening questionnaires in other cultures, such as the SRQ and GHQ-12 in Brazil (Mari & Williams, 1985, 1986). Based on the sensitivity and specificity coefficients for different cut-off scores, a cut-off score of 7–8 is recommended for epidemiological studies for the detection of CMD.

Relationship between emic and etic criteria of CMD

In the SSQ Study, the emic criterion of caseness was the clinical judgment of the care provider concerned and the etic criterion was the score on the CISR. Prevalence of CMD was over 50% on both criteria. Although kappa values of agreement between emic and etic criteria were low, the level of agreement of about 55% was higher than in other studies of care provider recognition of mental disorder, when an etic instrument was the criterion of caseness (reviewed in the first chapter).

Emic and etic criteria may disagree because of poor sensitivity and specificity of either set of criteria or because of a methodological artifact. In the SSQ Study, the care provider was more likely to classify patients as suffering from mental disorder than the CISR and the difference was particularly marked for TMP. An analysis of the patient variables associated with caseness (Patel & Mann, 1997) showed that of those participants whom care providers but not the CISR judged as cases (i.e. group 2 in Table 3.12), most were unemployed, poorly educated, and female. These patients were more likely to suffer from a chronic health problem and many considered a supernatural aetiology to their illness. These patients' problems were often assessed by care providers to have a psychosocial cause (by nurses and TMPs) or supernatural cause (by TMPs only). These observations suggest that many of these individuals had suffered an adverse social event and supernatural explanations were used to make these experiences meaningful. Because the care provider clinical judgment used in this study (adapted from that used in the WHO studies) classified all health problems as being either physical or mental with no social or supernatural categories, care providers may have been forced to indicate a mental disorder as a diagnosis of exclusion of physical disorder. Thus these patients, many of whom suffered longstanding social problems, were not mentally ill as per etic criteria. This hypothesis was supported by the finding that these mismatched patients had SSQ and positive mental health scores almost identical to group 1 in Table 3.12 (i.e. definite non-cases). Thus, a proportion of care provider "false–positives" may have been accounted for by an artifact of classification. Participants whom the CISR, but not the care provider, classified as cases (group 3 in Table 3.12) were more likely to be employed, have an acute problem and to consider *kufungisisa* as a cause of their problem. These participants had positive mental health scores similar to the definite cases. Their scores on the SSQ were also high, though lower than the cases, suggesting that they were moderately symptomatic participants. This group may then be a group of patients with CMD who were not recognised by care providers partly because they were marginally less symptomatic and because they presented with acute complaints (Patel & Mann, 1997).

RELEVANCE OF INDIGENOUS MODELS OF MENTAL ILLNESS

Concepts of mental illness

The Ethnographic Study aimed to elicit the concepts of CMD as held by a diverse group of carers in formal, traditional, and home-based caring situations (Patel et al., 1995a). The participants of the FGD reflected the realities of medical pluralism in Harare. The interview format included both open-ended questions about the nature and type of mental disorders and the views about the nature of the disorders in three case vignettes describing typical presentations of CMD. A key finding was that mental illness was most commonly associated with behavioural disturbances; thus, a person was recognised to suffer from a mental illness when his behaviour changed and when he was unable to look after himself or his family in the way he used to. Although the mind was sited in the head region, the soul and heart also played an important role in the mediation of emotions and behaviour, suggesting that inquiring about whether a patient believes his distress was related to the heart or soul could be a useful way of identifying mental illness. The types of mental illness were intimately related to beliefs about supernatural causation. Ancestral spirits guarded the traditions of society, and if these were broken in any way, the spirits could show their displeasure by inflicting illness. Evil spirits could be used by jealous persons to inflict illness. Beliefs in witchcraft were very much in evidence to explain misfortune. In addition to *kupenga* ("madness"), a variety of other types of mental illnesses were recognised, such as *mamhepo*, *kufungisisa*, *kutando botso*, *mhengeramumba*, and epilepsy. While some of these categories bore a phenomenological resemblance to biomedical categories (*kupenga* and acute psychoses; *kufungisisa* and CMD), others were related to specific situations such as breaking a particular type of taboo (for example, *kutanda botso*).

A variety of symptoms were elicited, the most prominent ones being behavioural disturbances and impairment of self-care. Cognitive, mood, and perceptual symptoms were of less importance. The frequency of somatic presentations was noted by nurses as being, at least in part, due to the social stigma of mental illness in the community. The greatest impact of mental illness was on the families of patients who not only bore the burden of caring for the patient and all financial expenses involved, but were also ostracised and isolated. Mentally ill persons were unlikely to find jobs and their marital life was likely to be severely affected by their aggressive and disinhibited behaviour. Both biomedical carers and TMPs could help mentally ill persons, depending on the cause of the illness, but often persons would consult both types of health care providers to resolve different issues relating to the same illness episode.

The case vignettes of CMD were recognised by the care providers in their communities. However, many felt that the descriptions did not reflect "illnesses", but social or spiritual problems associated with poverty, poor marital relationships and so on, and that, accordingly, the treatment for these were social, rather than medical. In describing the Igbo illness beliefs in Nigeria, Nzewi (1989) states that "a depressed individual is usually not considered mentally ill, particularly if there is a situational, precipitating factor...it is far more natural for the individual to react to misfortune by drifting into depression than not to react at all." Similarly, amongst the Yoruba, while emotional phenomena associated with neurotic disorders were recognised as distress states for which TMPs have cures, they were not labelled as mental illnesses (Murphy, 1976). In the sense that TMPs are also social workers in their communities, it was not surprising that they were seen as being important sources of care for all three vignettes.

Thus, other than the community psychiatric nurses, all the carers held on to traditional views of mental illness, a finding consistent with other studies from Africa (Abiodun, 1991). This is evidence that irrespective of the pace of "modernization" and formal education, traditional beliefs about illness and misfortune were unlikely to be replaced entirely by biomedical beliefs. Instead, new health concepts, such as AIDS and depression, were likely to be incorporated into the matrix of traditional concepts and a coherent whole rather than two distinct models would be used by patients and their families and care providers in response to illness and misfortune. Furthermore, it was evident that beliefs about causation guided the health-seeking behaviour of patients. With mental illness often being related to a supernatural cause, consulting traditional healers and *profitas* was a natural course of action. Although illness categories which psychiatry included under the rubric of CMD were recognised as being distressing and abnormal by care providers, these disorders were rarely considered as "mental" disorders. There was no equivalent term in Shona for "depression" or "anxiety". The term for mental illness, *kupenga*, dealt mainly with severe mental disorders. Using terms such as *kufungisisa* and supernatural disorders could convey the conceptually equivalent meaning of CMD (Patel et al., 1995a). Indeed, it is perhaps fortuitous that, given the social stigma attached to severe mental disorders, that CMD are not bracketed in the same category.

Explanatory models of patients with common mental disorders

The Phenomenology Study aimed to investigate the explanatory models and phenomenology of primary care attenders with conspicuous psychiatric morbidity as identified by their health care providers (Patel et al., 1995d). The principal objectives were to elicit indigenous constructs and symptoms of CMD. The former could then be compared to psychiatric concepts in the SSQ Study, while the latter would form the emic items of an indigenous psychiatric questionnaire (these were discussed in the previous section).

The illness was often chronic in duration. The chronicity of the illness may have reflected the selection bias of the care providers; thus, patients with acute somatic presentations were more likely to be considered to be suffering from a somatic illness, whereas those with repeated or long-standing complaints were considered to suffer from a mental disorder (and were therefore selected for the study). TMP attenders were more chronic, suggesting that patients consulted TMPs later in the course of their illness. This suggestion was supported by findings of a study on pathways to care (Patel, Simunyu, & Gwanzura, 1997a). Supernatural factors were the most frequently cited causes in response to open questions about causality. TMP attenders were more likely to consider supernatural causes; since patients had been interviewed after their consultation, it is possible that their models of illness had been influenced by the care provider. The other possibility was that patients' models of illness influence their health care provider seeking behaviour; this can only be clarified by a prospective study. When asked closed questions about specific causes, *kufungisisa* was admitted by 80% of patients. The illness was perceived as being severe with two-thirds reporting that they were unable to complete their daily activities on account of the illness. The main impact of the illness was on the ability to perform the necessary daily chores, whether they were household chores or occupational tasks.

Kufungisisa and psychiatric morbidity

Sociocultural factors play a profound role in the manifestation of CMD and indigenous idioms and concepts of illness need to be understood and related to biomedical psychiatric concepts originating in Euro-American cultures. Elucidating such concepts may be crucial in improving the understanding and recognition of mental illness and is one of the cornerstones of a culturally sensitive psychiatry. In the earlier two studies, the causal idioms of *kufungisisa* and supernatural problems, particularly witchcraft, were frequently linked to CMD. The relationship of both causal models with psychiatric morbidity were examined in the SSQ Study.

Kufungisisa was identified as one of two common complaints (the other being "a painful heavy heart") which were frequently associated with depression in a community sample of women in Harare (Abas et al., 1994). Studies in this book show that this term was used to describe both a concept or causal model of misfortune and illness, as well as an idiom of distress, i.e. a symptom of illness. In this sense, parallels can be drawn with the term "depression". Thus, *kufungisisa* can cause illness, and *kufungisisa* can be a symptom of illness. Conceptually, *kufungisisa* was related to worry and is consistent with Gelfand's early reports (1964) that severe worry was recognised as a cause of mental breakdown. Those patients who considered *kufungisisa* as a cause were more likely to feel that their illness had an emotional component and were more likely to consider supernatural causes for their illness. This latter finding is at odds with the suggestion that *kufungisisa* is different from "madness" in that the latter was viewed as being caused by "witchcraft and spirit possession" (Abas et al., 1994). Supernatural models of illness causation are widely held by the Shona community and care providers (Bourdillon, 1987; Patel et al., 1995a) and much misfortune can be traced to these roots. Indeed, patients who felt *kufungisisa* was causing their illness were *more likely* to consider spiritual or supernatural causes than other patients. When idioms of distress were related to the concept of *kufungisisa*, the constellation of idioms straddles the biomedical categories of anxiety and depression. The prominent idioms were worrying about life's problems (in particular, socioeconomic and marital problems), worrying about one's health, becoming forgetful, losing interest in social interactions, and being easily startled or panicky. Somatic symptoms included tiredness, palpitations, headache, pains in the side, and abdominal discomfort. The severity of morbidity of nonpsychotic psychological symptoms was higher in *kufungisisa* patients on two measures of psychiatric morbidity, the SSQ and CISR. Such patients were also more likely to be classified as cases on four sets of case criteria. Thus, the indigenous causal model of *kufungisisa* was strongly related to CMD on a range of measures (Patel, Simunyu, & Gwanzura, 1995c).

The concept of "thinking too much" has been reported from other African countries such as Nigeria, South Africa, Malawi, Ethiopia and Kenya (Cheetham & Cheetham, 1976; Good, 1987; Kortmann, 1987; Odejide et al., 1977; Peltzer, 1989). Some authors have suggested that vague complaints such as "too much thinking" may partly account for the low recognition of depression and anxiety (Pretorius, 1995). Of interest is the reporting of this construct from non-African societies as well. For example, *koucharang* is the Cambodian term for thinking too much and has been described as a culture-bound stress-related syndrome characterised by somatic complaints and behavioural changes (Frye & D'Avanzo, 1994). Conceptually similar constructs can be identified in other cultures; for example "nerves" is a term used to describe a general neurotic spectrum of distress states in Latin American societies; Nations, Camino, and Walker (1988) have shown that this idiom is related to anxiety and depression, is commoner in women, and tends to occur in association with negative life events. The issue of whether these indigenous constructs are simply local terms for what is "really" a depressive or anxiety disorder remains unresolved and, as far as some authors are concerned, irrelevant. Thus, Makanjuola (1987), while describing the condition *ode ori* in Nigeria, states that although there may be symptoms of anxiety and depression it is not unlikely that these are secondary to the "real" disorder of *ode ori*!

Supernatural causation and psychiatric morbidity

Murdock, Wilson, and Frederick's (1980) models of aetiology, based on a worldwide survey, classified illness into two basic groups: (1) theories of natural causation, such as infections, accidents and organic deterioration; and (2) theories of supernatural causation, which included mystical causes (e.g. fate, ominous sensations, contagion, mystical retribution), animistic causation (e.g. soul loss, spirit aggression), and magical causation (e.g. witchcraft and sorcery). While this twofold classification has been criticised on the grounds that human agencies such as sorcery are lumped together with nonhuman agencies such as spirits, the framework serves as a useful starting point to investigate the relationship between supernatural causes and mental illness not least because the subcategories of the former are often intricately interlinked and patients may carry both explanatory models of their illness causation (Eisenbruch, 1990). Beliefs in supernatural causation of illness is one of the most widespread explanatory models of mental illness in Africa.

Although patients from the SSQ Study who held a supernatural causal model were more likely to be present in the TMP sample, it is notable that more than a quarter of PHC attenders also held this view. While the diagnosis of the health care provider plays some role in moulding a patient's explanatory model of illness, it is not necessarily the most important influence (Hunt et al., 1989); this may account for the relatively high proportion of patients who subscribe to the supernatural model in the PHC sample. Furthermore, it is likely that the PHC figure is an underestimate, because of the bias introduced by virtue of being interviewed in a biomedical facility by a biomedical researcher. Supernatural causal labels used by patients were most commonly *chivanhu* (traditional African problem), being bewitched, and *mamhepo* (bad airs). All three labels are essentially magical (as opposed to animistic or mystical). Patients who had a supernatural causal model were less educated, more likely to be unemployed, and to suffer a chronic illness. Such patients were more likely to present with psychosocial complaints, to consider *kufungisisa* as an associated cause for their illness, and to consider that the illness involved their mind or soul. It was interesting to note that belief in supernatural causes was not related to religious affiliation, since Christianity (the commonest denomination in Zimbabwe) officially rejects the notion of a spirit world. This finding is consistent with ethnographic data suggesting that many indigenous Zimbabweans hold on to both Christian and traditional beliefs without much conflict (Bourdillon, 1987) and that many consider supernatural models to explain illness and misfortune (Chavunduka, 1978). Patients with supernatural distress scored higher on the two measures of nonpsychotic mental disorder, the SSQ and CISR, the difference being statistically significant for the SSQ score. Such patients were more likely to be classified as cases on three of four case criteria. Six Shona idioms found to predict supernatural distress resemble the biomedical construct of anxiety. Four idioms were cognitive with worry and panic being the core features, while two idioms were somatic symptoms reported in other phenomenological studies of mental disorder in Africa (Awaritefe, 1988; Ihezue, 1989; Jegede, 1979; Makanjuola, 1987; Peltzer, 1989). Thus, the supernatural causal model, in particular related to witchcraft, is associated with the biomedical construct of CMD and may be related more specifically to the construct of anxiety (Patel, 1995b): whether the supernatural model is used to explain the distressing symptoms of nonpsychotic mental illness or whether the supernatural factors cause the symptoms is related to the theoretical model of illness causation. Thus the latter hypothesis cannot be valid from the biomedical standpoint, while it is valid from the theory of traditional medicine.

There is evidence to suggest that the type of causal model may have some specificity in relation to the type of mental illness. For example, a

Nigerian study reported that neurotic patients were more likely to adduce supernatural explanations as compared to psychosocial explanations used by psychotic patients (Ilechukwu, 1988). Differentiation between animistic (i.e. spiritual) and magical theories (e.g. witchcraft) has been examined by some authors. A study from South Africa with 100 Zulu psychiatric patients showed that, although both psychoses and neuroses were associated with supernatural causes, magical causes were more likely to be associated with neurotic disorders while animistic causes were associated with psychotic disorders (Edwards et al., 1983). These findings suggest that there may be an interaction between the nature of a misfortune and the explanation given to it and that such illness attributions are not simply random findings (Swartz, 1986). The stigma attached to mental illness is partly due to the belief that that it may be the fault of the individual or family (Obot, 1989) which ties in with the findings that psychotic disorders are often conceptualised as being the result of breaking of social taboos and angering the ancestral spirits. In contrast, neurotic disorders are the result of witchcraft and this externalises the cause of distress and reduces individual responsibility and, thus, the associated stigma. According to some authors, the stigma of psychiatric consultation carries a greater labelling potential than the transient crisis of spirit possession (Lefley, 1984). This model would also explain why neurotic disorders are rarely conceptualised as being psychiatric problems.

Witchcraft plays a central role in African cosmology; the core of this belief system is that witches can do harm from a distance without being in physical contact with the victim (Binitie, 1991). There have been many negative connotations attached to beliefs in witchcraft, not least their potential role of dividing communities and the not uncommon lethal consequences of "outing" a witch. Althought witchcraft is officially outlawed in Zimbabwe and open accusations of identifying purported witches are rare nowadays, beliefs in witchcraft remain widespread. Some authors have argued that this belief system plays an important role in defining the contexts of social strains and stresses and that even accusations may function in the role of social control. According to Chavunduka (1982), the suggestion that the "solution" to witchcraft is to encourage people to abandon their beliefs in it is as "senseless" as telling a physician that he could eradicate malaria merely by denying its existence.

From a clinical perspective, beliefs in supernatural causation of CMD may have considerable therapeutic implications. Studies on the outcome of psychotherapy have shown that patients with a psychological model of illness are more likely to be compliant with psychotherapy and have an improved outcome, suggesting that congruence of patient and care provider explanatory models is a key factor in outcome (Foulks, Persons,

& Merkel, 1986). The corollary may hold true for supernatural causal models. For example, in Madagascar, TMPs were reported to be more successful with patients with spirit possession since they accepted and transformed patients' explanations for their experiences as compared to psychiatrists who were unable to understand these experiences due to their acceptance of a cognitive model based on Euro-American sensibilities (Sharp, 1994). Within the biomedical setting, beliefs in witchcraft are likely to appear in the course of psychotherapy with patients from cultures which believe in supernatural causation and by allowing a patient to ventilate freely these concerns may open up new therapeutic avenues (Neki et al., 1986). Indeed, eliciting spiritual and religious beliefs should be an integral part of the routine psychiatric assessment not only since they may assist in improving communication with the patient but may also help predict outcome (Sims, 1994). At the primary care level, incorporating local concepts such as supernatural models in the training of primary health care providers may help improve the recognition of nonpsychotic mental illness (Patel & Winston, 1994).

EPIDEMIOLOGY OF COMMON MENTAL DISORDERS

Prevalence of psychiatric morbidity in PHC and TMP attenders

The hypothesis that the prevalence of psychiatric morbidity was greater in TMP as compared to PHC attenders was found to be true on three of four case criteria used. Just over a quarter of attenders at PHCs were found to be cases of CMD (as judged by the gold standard used in the study). This figure is higher than the 10% rate reported in a Zimbabwean study from the mid-1980s (Hall & Williams, 1987) but similar to the 26% reported recently by Reeler et al. (1993). This suggests a rising prevalence of CMD which is not implausible, given the worsening socioeconomic conditions in Zimbabwe since 1987. Further, there is growing evidence suggesting an association between acculturation and urbanisation in low-income countries and higher rates of mental disorder (Harpham, 1994) and both these processes are typical of the changes in contemporary Zimbabwean society.

Nearly 40% of TMP attenders were found to be cases; there are no comparable studies published from Africa. However, this finding is consistent with anecdotal evidence suggesting that a substantial proportion of TMP attenders suffer from CMD (de Jong, 1987; Edgerton, 1980; Gelfand et al., 1985; Harding, 1975; Jahoda, 1961; Peltzer, 1988; Staugard, 1985). Indeed, some authors have stated that it is fortuitous that TMPs can fill in the role of helping such patients since the number of mental health professionals in Africa is woefully inadequate (Lamont, 1988).

Furthermore, TMPs by virtue of understanding the cultural norms of their patients, and in particular by being conversant with the ritual treatments of supernatural causes, may be more effective therapists for CMD. The potential role of the TMP in mental health care is discussed later.

The Case–Control Study

This study is the first Case–Control Study examining the associations of CMD in primary care settings in Africa to employ an indigenously developed case finding questionnaire and to sample attenders for three principal types of primary health care providers, viz. primary health clinics, general practitioners, and traditional medical practitioners.

Target sample sizes were recruited without difficulty, and the non-response rate was low (4%). Most of the nonrespondents were GP attenders and the reasons they gave for not being able to take part in the study were because they were employed and unable to take time off for the interviews. The differences in the samples of each group recruited from the different care provider types were consistent with the nature of health seeking behaviour in Harare. Thus, those attending GPs had higher incomes than TMP and PHC attenders, reflecting the fee structures of these care providers and the fact that many were in full-time employment which provided private medical insurance cover. TMP attenders were more likely to be unemployed and to suffer a chronic illness. Since the study involved prevalent cases it is not possible to ascertain the extent to which an association preexisted development of CMD and could be of aetiological significance.

From this study we are able to build a picture of the characteristics of patients with CMD who were attending a primary health care service in Harare. Such a person was more likely to be a woman from a large family (i.e. with many children), although in a small but statistically significant group, infertility was an important factor. Associations of female gender with CMD have ranged from a negative association in Ibadan (OR 0.3) to a positive association in Bangalore (OR 1.9) in the WHO study (Goldberg & Lecrubier, 1995); the latter is similar to our findings. While some of this variability may be accounted for by varying patterns of health seeking in different cultures (since all data are primary care rather than community), it is also possible that actual rates of disorder may vary according to sociocultural factors such as the role of women in society, their social support structures, and the unique stresses they may face. Patients of either sex with CMD typically presented with three or more somatic symptoms of greater than one-month duration. They were more likely to be under acute economic stress having recently lost a job, having no cash savings, and having been unable to buy food in the previous month due to lack of money. These findings are resonant with the strong associations of poor economic status and CMD in industrialised societies. The association of caseness with unemployment is one that has also been reported in the WHO multinational study although, as with gender, the association is highly variable across the 14 study sites (Goldberg & Lecrubier, 1995). Alcohol use was not associated with CMD.

The explanatory models of illness show those with a CMD were more likely to consider a psychosocial cause for their illness (e.g. "poverty", "thinking too much"). They were also more likely to consider witchcraft and *kufungisisa* as causes of their distress, replicating the findings of the SSQ Study. Although many admitted to a history of stress, it was evident that the meaning of stress often reflected socioeconomic and family problems which were also reported by a substantial proportion of those without a CMD. The life events checklist used had been found to be of value in earlier studies in Zimbabwe and was felt to be of sufficient value to determine simple associations with specific events and difficulties over the previous year. The two most prominent associations were with infertility and loss of job. The former is of particular interest, since almost 10% of cases had experienced difficulties in having children, and yet just one participant was recognised as having an infertility problem by care providers. One of the crucial social roles of a married or cohabiting couple in traditional African societies is having children and the failure to conceive may play an important role as a stressor and precipitant for CMD. The protective effect of childbirth for men may reflect the differing cultural context of this event for the two sexes. This association is particularly important since infertility may not only lead to emotional problems, but the latter are recognised as a cause of infertility as well. These findings underline the cultural context of the role of life difficulties, the importance of primary health workers recognising infertility, and the need for appropriate referral.

CMD causes considerable disruption of daily life and was associated with a perception of a poor quality of life which is consistent with other studies (Ormel et al., 1994, 1993). Cases spent almost twice the number of days unable to work or bedridden in the month prior to interview. We evaluated the comorbidity of physical illness by asking GPs and nurses to record their primary diagnoses and current treatments (from the medical cards and their current consultation). Since many patients never saw a doctor in the PHC, medical diagnoses as recorded on case notes were not always definitive or reliable. However, the method of assessing physical disorder was considered in some detail at the outset of the study and a practical, cost-effective and reliable way of determining the presence and nature of a physical illness could not be identified. The only method which was considered reliable was a detailed physical examination. However, not only would this have required a number of medically qualified staff who were already in short supply in the high-density suburbs, such an examination would have not ruled out the commonest causes of physical illness such as chronic infectious and diarrheal diseases. Biochemical and pathological investigations were not availabe in the PHCs and the logistics and expense of such investigations precluded their use. Furthermore, neither physical nor pathological examinations would have been practical for TMP attenders. Despite the high prevalence of HIV disease in Zimbabwe, we were not able to examine the relationship between this disease and CMD for reasons of ethics and confidentiality. It is likely that HIV disease with its implications of increasing mortality rates amongst younger adults and consequent bereavements and breakdown of family structure leads to CMD. This is a topic which urgently deserves research attention, not just in Zimbabwe but in many African and Asian countries where HIV is a growing public health problem. No attempt was made to imply that the prevalence figures of CMD reflected the absence or severity of a coexisting physical illness. Physical illness diagnoses (for PHC and GP attenders) did not differ between cases and controls, suggesting that disability was probably associated with CMD itself although it is possible that part of this association may be accounted for by the greater severity of a coexisting physical illness in those with a CMD.

TMP attenders had a chronic illness as compared to PHC and GP attenders and over 80% of both groups consulted a biomedical carer first. Both findings are evidence of the cultural belief that much illness, when acute, is considered to be physical or natural, and biomedicine is perceived to be more effective than traditional medicine; it is only when an illness becomes chronic that a reevaluation of the causal model occurs and TMPs are consulted (Chavunduka, 1978; Patel et al., 1997a). Cases were more likely to have consulted a TMP or a church-based priest or pastor in the previous year. This finding may be related to the association of caseness with chronicity and with the belief in being a victim of witchcraft suggesting that, as an illness became chronic, patients used culturally meaningful modes of explaining and responding to their distress. Indeed, an examination of the data showed a strong association between chronicity and beliefs in witchcraft. Those who had a belief in witchcraft were more likely to have chronic illness (71% vs. 37%, OR 4.2, 95% CI 2.4–7.1).

PHC nurses and GPs were more likely to identify a mental disorder in cases, recognising up to a fifth of the morbidity which is at the midpoint of rates published in earlier studies in Zimbabwe (Hall & Williams, 1987) and the SSQ Study in this book. This variation suggests that recognition rates are dependent on a range of variables, including site- and carer-specific factors such as their concepts of mental illness. TMPs used the causal labels of *kufungisisa* and witchcraft more often for cases, which resonates with the causal models held by patients themselves. These findings further confirm the suggestions that indigenous models are closely related to CMD and could be used in training programmes for the community and health workers to improve the awareness and recognition of CMD. Despite the growing evidence of the efficacy of antidepressants in the management of CMD (e.g. Mynors-Wallis, Gath, Lloyd-Thomas, & Tomlinson, 1995), it was notable that these drugs were never prescribed by the PHC staff and rarely so by the GP; the commonest treatments were symptomatic drugs and there was a trend for cases to receive benzodiazepines and injectable drugs.

DIRECTIONS FOR FUTURE RESEARCH

Psychiatric epidemiology in Sub-Saharan Africa has been mostly etic in nature, using instruments and diagnostic models devised in Euro-American cultures. Despite these limitations, research has demonstrated a high prevalence of psychiatric morbidity in community and primary care settings. Ethnographic research has revealed a range of causal beliefs and types of mental illnesses in Africa and showed that neurotic disorders are rarely recognised as mental disorders by the community. The principal limitation of the emic approach has been the lack of reliability and a link with practical issues related to mental health services. The "new" cross-cultural psychiatry proposed that the integration of etic and emic approaches was required to enable a culture sensitive psychiatric model which was also comparable across cultures to emerge.

The research described in this monograph has been influenced by the theory of the "new" cross-cultural psychiatry in the following ways: incorporating ethnographic data to determine constructs of illness which approximate biomedical concepts of CMD; eliciting the explanatory models of patients with conspicuous psychiatric morbidity, i.e. cases of mental disorder identified by primary care providers; eliciting of idioms of distress of patients with conspicuous psychiatric morbidity; using bilingual trained personnel with ongoing monitoring rather than interpreters during the interview process; devising a case finding questionnaire based on those indigenous idioms and etic symptoms which best predicted CMD; using a gold standard of caseness which required agreement between etic and emic criteria; involvement of TMPs and TMP attenders in all stages of the study; basing of the study in primary care rather than hospital psychiatric populations; examining the relationship between indigenous constructs of mental disorder and biomedical constructs; and attempting to link ethnographic and descriptive research with practical clinical epidemiology by conducting the Case–Control Study and a 12-month follow-up study which has been recently completed (Patel et al., 1997d).

Cross-cultural psychiatry has been described as a "jungle of speculation but a desert of information; it is a subject which promises to illuminate the social determinants of psychiatric disorder but this promise is unlikely to be fulfilled until the social characteristics of the culture is specified, the hypotheses carefully focused, and funds forthcoming to support such studies" (Bebbington, 1993). These recommendations are important not only for furthering the knowledge of the nature of human psychological suffering, but also to facilitate communication with health workers in low-income countries and to determine the effective ways of caring for persons with a CMD.

Health–systems research (HSR) in low-income countries

Research in low-income regions should follow the principles of HSR whose emphasis lies in solving problems which are relevant to the priorities of local health care workers and whose methodologies are mainly influenced by local sociocultural factors (Abas et al., 1994; Chandiwana, 1992). Research of this nature would not only have the potential of bringing about useful and sustainable change but would also fulfill academic needs. HSR poses a theoretical challenge to the notion of cross-cultural psychiatry itself; if biomedical psychiatry is a product of Euro-American culture, then all psychiatric research is by definition "cross-cultural", thus rendering the term redundant. HSR offers a more useful and pragmatic approach in its recognition that the key influences on mental illness are the complex interactions between biology and the social, economic, cultural, and political environments in different regions of the world.

A fundamental goal of HSR is to facilitate communication between health care workers and patients. Cross-cultural research is fraught with innumerable difficulties, communication being the first and most obvious (Cheetham & Rzadkowolski, 1980). Communication in psychiatric research must include dissemination of information back to the communities from where data were collected; Lin (1983) argues that psychiatric research appears to use the people and societies of less developed countries as objects or samples of study for their own scientific interest without feeding the results back. Communication which patients understand and is within their sphere of social and cultural contexts can lead to improved compliance and better patient satisfaction (Ley, 1988). Communication at primary care level requires an understanding of patient explanatory models, since simple agreement of diagnostic label of a patient's condition may be no guarantee for agreement on its aetiology or treatment and, on the contrary, may provide a false impression of consensus (Helman, 1985). A key issue in communication with patients and primary care providers is the concept of neuroses. This gap in communication is perhaps best exemplified by a personal experience. In 1993, a depression education programme was undertaken on the basis of the guidelines suggested by the depression research studies conducted in 1992 (Abas et al., 1994). This programme included educating nurses on the signs and symptoms of depression, use of a multiple symptom card, counselling skills, and problem solving. However, in the year of the education programme, the total number of registered cases of psychiatric illness was only 933 which represented just 0.001% of new attenders (City of Harare Health Department, 1994). This figure was no different from that of 1992 and showed a very low level of recognition, particularly when compared to prevalence statistics for CMD in Zimbabwe. Reasons given by nurses to explain the low recorded rates at a follow-up workshop were: discomfort in recording such distress as a mental illness since many patients only needed "a bit of counselling" and were not "really mentally ill"; the perception that the serious physical illness and social problems facing patients made their emotional distress "under-standable" and unlikely to respond to psychological interventions; the concern that a psychiatric label was stigmatising and could alienate patients from continuing treatment; and the concern that a psychiatric diagnosis could lead to an increase in the workload of the few CPN in the city (Patel, 1996). Thus, rather than lack of awareness, there appeared to be a conceptual divide between the models of depression in psychiatry and primary health care.

Neurotic disorders occur all over the world; they represent a universal human experience in response to adversity and loss. However, this does not imply that their clinical subcategories are universally valid, or even that their rightful place in the medical lexicon is under the psychiatric pigeon-hole. CMDs are not as conspicuous in low-income countries because sufferers do not perceive themselves as mentally disturbed, nor do health workers consider them as such (Giel, 1982). CMD probably represent a biologically determined final common pathway in the human response to loss, defeat, or demoralisation; however, the cultural concept of the person influences the psychopathological process both by determining the individual cognitive representation of self and by regulating interpersonal behaviour in a fashion that amplifies or moderates dysphoric mood (Kirmayer, 1989). Evidence from the studies in this monograph suggest that future research should move away from the psychiatric oriented perspectives that dominate current conceptualisation of CMD in favour of a language more easily understood by nonspecialists.

The use of broad terms such as "neurasthenia" in China or *kufungisisa* in Zimbabwe is a practical approach to this conceptual–semantic problem.

In most African countries, medical students mainly encounter psychotic illness during their psychiatric training, rendering classroom teaching on CMD theoretical and unrelated to a real clinical problem. Thus, the teaching of the nature, diagnosis, and management of CMD could be rooted in the subject discipline of community or primary care medicine as a reflection of the characteristic clinical setting of CMD (Patel, 1996). Alternative methods of training and management of mental health problems such as the use of behaviourally determined, atheoretical, and pragmatic categories which form part of a problem-oriented approach may be more effective than a psychiatric biomedical model (Essex & Gosling, 1983). Psychiatrists in Africa are largely concerned with the care of psychotic patients, particularly those who are acutely ill and showing disturbed behaviour (Asuni, 1991; Ben-Tovim & Boyce, 1988). There are few psychiatrists, most of whom have trained overseas and in the ICD/DSM model. Thus, reliance on them as the sole experts for problems in primary care risks reaffirming the universals of psychiatry and rendering communication with primary care staff and the community more difficult. Studies must therefore involve PHC staff and TMP in order to be representative of the local culture. There needs to be greater involvement of private GPs who are key providers of family health care in many low-income countries. Research must be multidisciplinary with active involvement of development agencies and nongovernmental organisations (Patel, Mutambirwa, & Nhiwatiwa, 1995b). The latter now play a major role in health service development and research in many African and other low-income countries. Despite often focusing on populations at the greatest risk for CMD, for example women, refugees and the poor, rarely does mental health receive any attention. In the author's view, this is a symptom of the lack of dialogue on practical mental health issues between psychiatry and its partners in health care. Arguably, the biggest limitation in the current approach to multinational studies is the assumption that psychiatric research can be conducted free from adaptation for local social, political, economic, and health service circumstances.

Culture and the treatment of CMD

A key area for future research is the examination of the role of culture in the management, treatment response, and outcome of CMD. Despite a general consensus in psychiatry about the effectiveness of antidepressants for CMD in primary care (Paykel & Priest, 1992), it is surprising to note that there are no published randomised controlled trials evaluating the efficacy of antidepressants in primary care from low-income countries.

While it may be felt that cultural factors are unlikely to influence treatment response for physical treatments such as antidepressants, there is evidence suggesting that the effective dose of antidepressants is lower amongst non-Causasians (Marsella & Westermeyer, 1993); an open trial in Kenya showed that 75mgs of clomipramine daily was as effective as 150mgs (Kilonzo et al., 1994). The cultural component is likely to be even greater for psychotherapeutic interventions. Clinical evidence suggests that conventional Euro-American models of psychotherapy with their orientation towards individuality and intrapsychic introspection are of limited efficacy with neurotic problems in African patients (Cheetham & Griffiths, 1980, 1982; Swartz, 1987). In Africa, psychotherapy in mental health settings is often superficial; reliance is mainly on drugs and ECT. Nevertheless, there is still scope to adapt and evaluate brief psychological interventions, particularly those which emphasise the "here and now" aspects of ill health such as problem solving for use in low-income countries. Potential themes for research include adapting psychological treatments for use in different cultures, for example by incorporating local constructs of illness such as supernatural causal models. Regional factors such as costs of antidepressants and the availability of personnel for psychological interventions are likely to play an equally important role in influencing the practical aspects of implementation of a treatment strategy. Thus, it is essential that randomised controlled trials of antidepressant and brief psychological interventions are undertaken in low-income countries to confirm their efficacy and cost effectiveness in these settings.

Traditional treatments which are symbolically similar to psychotherapies may be a fruitful alternative to the management of CMD, for example by offering spiritual treatments for victims of witchcraft (Asuni, 1991; Cheetham & Griffiths, 1982). The combination of widespread use of healers and the problems with health manpower highlights the need for innovative experiments in making healers copartners in primary health care. There is resistance to such a move from two influential sectors of society. First, there is a wide gulf between orthodox Christian and traditional religion and the former are one of the principal sponsors of biomedical health care in the country. Traditional medicine has its roots in traditional religion which has an extensive and rich belief system in spirits. These beliefs were shunned as being pagan and primitive by Christian missionairies who, in an effort to convert people to Christianity, devalued traditional medicine and offered biomedical health care as an alternative (Bourdillon, 1987). Second, biomedical health practitioners, not least nurses, have grave doubts about traditional medicine. Thus, healers are accused of being backward, unscientific or static, although studies show that they have the ability to adapt to changing knowledge about medicine, for example, increasingly recognising that some illnesses respond better to biomedicine and referring such patients accordingly (Berger, 1995; Gelfand et al., 1985; Winston et al., 1995). Many healers are accused of being charlatans, a suspicion confirmed by some healers themselves; organisations such as ZINATHA are attempting to weed out such healers by the process of registration. There are concerns that traditional medicines are ineffective and may lead to potentially lethal delays in seeking appropriate medical care. Furthermore, concerns are expressed about the toxic side-effects of some traditional medicines (Nhachi & Kasilo, 1992). Those who support traditional medicine argue that the chronicity of TMP attenders means that such patients are likely to have a poorer prognosis anyway and that observations made in biomedical facilities miss out on patients who recovered with traditional medicine (Bourguignon, 1989; Heggenhougen & Sesia-Lewis, 1988). It has been argued that the two types of health professionals would not be able to work together. However, recent work has shown that although there is initial mistrust, collaboration is not only possible, but effective (Hoff & Nhlavana Maseko, 1986). In a pilot study in Zimbabwe involving cooperation between traditional and biomedical healers, patients reported that they were very satisfied with being able to consult both, and asked why this was not more widely available (Stott et al., 1988). The experiences of the author with TMPs in Harare has been unequivocally one of open cooperation and participation with a keen willingness not only to inform about their theories and beliefs but to listen to and accept those of biomedicine.

Anecdotal evidence suggests that traditional medicine may be of benefit to specific groups of patients, especially those with psychosocial problems. Indeed, the skills of TMP in the management of mental illness are recognised not only by themselves (Fanuel, 1992), but the biomedical sector as well (Chikara & Manley, 1991; Jilek, 1993; Makanjuola & Jaiyeola, 1987; Mossop & Stratford, 1986; Wessels, 1985). A follow-up of cases with CMD by the author and colleagues in Zimbabwe has produced the first epidemiological evidence that recognition of caseness by TMPs leads to an improved outcome (Patel et al., 1997d). However, there is little other objective research demonstrating the efficacy of traditional treatments for health problems, leading some authors to argue that an integration of traditional and biomedicine is "wishful thinking" and to criticise anthropologists for their uncritical belief in the efficacy of TMP (Velimirovic, 1992).

There is an urgent need to formulate a framework for evaluating both biomedical and traditional treatments for CMD which closely involve both groups of health carers. Such research will need to be innovative in its methodology since orthodox study designs such as the randomised controlled trial are unlikely to be suitable for traditional medicine. Since treatment research in primary care in low-income countries is virtually nonexistent, the range of potential research themes is enormous. Some examples which are relevant to the findings presented in this book are: whether the congruence of explanatory models between patient and care provider influences outcome; whether open access to both biomedical and traditional treatments leads to a better outcome as opposed to the current system which is one of mutual exclusion by both groups of care providers; and whether the incorporation of indigenous constructs of illness into the training of biomedical health workers and the use of culturally sensitive screening questionnaires lead to higher recognition and improved outcome. Whilst prevention of CMD remains a complex issue, the identification of risk factors, such as the inability to buy food due to poverty and unemployment, suggests a link between hunger, retrenchment, poverty, psychological illness, health service use, and disability in a society which is already crippled by economic hardships (Logie & Woodroffe, 1993). Research could examine whether policy initiatives, for example to reduce hunger by food subsidies and to reduce the economic impact of unemployment, decrease the morbidity of CMD. Only such research will help clarify the roles of complementary medical systems and health and social policies in the prevention and treatment of CMD in Africa. Thus, an integrative health care policy and greater research with an interface between development and health is essential in Africa (Lambo, 1969; Ben-Tovim, 1987; Dauskardt, 1990).

CHAPTER FIVE

Conclusions

The studies described in this book are an attempt to integrate ethnographic and epidemiological research methods in a sequential project which described local models and factors associated with CMD in primary care settings in Harare, Zimbabwe. Since the studies were based in urban areas and were focused on primary care attenders, it is unlikely that the findings can be generalised to rural or community settings. However, the study has established a model for investigating psychiatric illness in a culturally sensitive way which can be adapted for use in these settings. The key conclusions of these studies is an evaluation of the influence of culture on CMD.

Despite modernisation and urbanisation, beliefs about the causes and types of mental illness are closely linked to traditional beliefs, in particular beliefs in the causal role of supernatural factors and *kufungisisa*. Although somatic symptoms are the commonest presenting complaints of CMD, the majority of patients with a CMD perceive that their illness has an emotional component. Thus somatic symptoms are an accompaniment rather than an alternative to the expression of CMD. A combination of idioms of distress derived from patient symptoms and items from biomedical questionnaires help predict CMD in a primary care population. The Shona Symptom Questionnaire is the first indigenously developed psychiatric measure of CMD in Africa which has incorporated idioms of distress of biomedical and traditional medical attenders. It has 14 items, most of which are nonsomatic. Perceptual disturbances are related to

CMD in this setting. However, it was also clear that most, if not all, of the 14 items are fairly universal in their character. Indeed, the shortened Shona version of the SRQ shares seven of its eight items with the SSQ; agreement of case classification between the SSQ and the SRQ exceeded 80% (Patel & Todd, 1996). Similarly, the patients' perceptions of the emotional nature of their illness showed, if anything, higher levels of agreement with biomedical criteria as compared to the judgment of their care providers. Thus, in the view of this author, the broad category of neuroses, or CMD, can be measured or detected equally well using either an etic instrument or an indigenously developed one. However, it is also clear from the SRQ study quoted above that it is imperative to ensure a conceptually equivalent translation and to reevaluate the validity and cut-off scores of etic instruments whenever used in new settings.

The broad concept of psychological distress encompassed under the rubric of CMD is recognised in the Shona culture. This agreement does not imply that the subcategories of CMD are valid, nor even that the rightful place of CMD is in the psychiatric pigeon-hole at all. CMD, though recognised by care providers as distress states, are rarely considered to be psychiatric disorders or as needing psychiatric treatment. Subcategories such as anxiety and depression cannot be conceptually translated into Shona and these symptoms are highly associated with one another, contradicting the categorical approach to their classification. Thus, psychiatric research needs to accept the clinical reality that CMD are rarely differentiated into numerous subcategories in primary care. The emphasis on complex classifications and developing lengthy interviews distracts attention from the practical issues of developing innovative approaches to tackling the huge problems of CMD in low-income countries and risks alienating psychiatric research from its partners in local health systems research. Indigenous causal models such as *kufungisisa* and supernatural causation are closely related to biomedical concepts of CMD and incorporating these in the training of health care workers may improve their recognition of CMD and communication with patients.

Up to half of TMP attenders and a third of PHC attenders suffer from a CMD. CMD in primary care attenders in urban Zimbabwe is strongly associated with female gender and economic impoverishment. Patients are more likely to have a chronic illness, to be disabled by their illness, and to be unemployed. A recently completed one-year follow-up of the cohort of cases recruited in the case–control study has shown that morbidity was persistent in 40% of the sample and that it remained significantly associated with disability (Patel et al, 1997d). Thus, CMD are not only very common, but they affect the most vulnerable and poorest sections of society and, in turn, disable them for long periods. Although the illness was recognised by health care providers in a proportion of cases, they were rarely given what psychiatry recognises as effective interventions such as antidepressant drugs or structured psychological interventions. The paucity of reliable outcome studies or trials of interventions in primary care from low-income countries may account for this apparent lack of effective interventions. This evidence points to an urgent need to bring CMD into the mainstream of community medicine and public health for it is only through these routes that there will be greater recognition of its public health implications. Perhaps here lies the single most important influence of culture on CMD: many cultures do not accept CMD in the same boat as severe mental disorders with its attendant stigmas. Instead of attempting to change the explanatory models of entire communities to come in line with those of a largely hospital based biomedical psychiatry, it would be more pragmatic to adapt the psychiatric approach to CMD to fit the models and beliefs already existing in the community.

References

Abas, M., Broadhead, J., Mbape, P., & Khumalo-Sakatukwa, G. (1994). Defeating depression in the developing world: A Zimbabwean model. *British Journal of Psychiatry, 164*, 293–296.

Abiodun, O.A. (1989). Psychiatric morbidity in a primary health care centre in a rural community in Nigeria. *Central African Journal of Medicine, 34*, 372–377.

Abiodun, O.A. (1991). Knowledge and attitude concerning mental health of primary health care workers in Nigeria. *International Journal of Social Psychiatry, 37*, 113–120.

Al-Issa, I. (1995). The illusion of reality or the reality of illusion: Hallucinations and culture. *British Journal of Psychiatry, 166*, 368–373.

American Psychiatric Association (1985). *Diagnostic and Statistical Manual* (3rd edn., rev.). Washington: APA.

Angst, J. (1973). Masked depression viewed from the cross-cultural standpoint. *International Symposium, St Moritz, (Abstract)* 269–274.

Araya, R., Robert, W., Richard, L., & Lewis, G. (1994). Psychiatric morbidity in primary health care in Santiago, Chile: Preliminary findings. *British Journal of Psychiatry, 165*, 530–532.

Asuni, T. (1991). Development of psychiatry in Africa. In S.O. Okpaku (Ed.), *Mental health in Africa and the Americas today* (p. 17). Nashville: Chrisolith Books.

Awaritefe, A. (1988). Clinical anxiety in Nigeria. *Acta Psychiatrica Scandinavica, 77*, 729–735.

Ayorinde, A. (1977). Heat in the head or body: A semantic confusion? *African Journal of Psychiatry, 1*, 59–63.

Baasher, T.A. (1982). Epidemiological surveys in developing countries. *Acta Psychiatrica Scandinavica, Suppl. 296, 65*, 45–51.

Babor, T.F., de la Fuente, J.R., Saunders, J., & Grant, M. (1992). *AUDIT: The Alcohol Use Disorders Identification Test*. Geneva: World Health Organisation.

Babor, T.F. & Grant, M. (1992). *Programme on substance abuse: Project on identification and management of alcohol related problems.* Geneva: World Health Organisation.

Baskin, D. (1984). Cross-cultural conceptions of mental illness. *Psychiatric Quarterly, 56,* 45–53.

Bebbington, P. (1993). Transcultural aspects of affective disorders. *International Review of Psychiatry, 5,* 145–156.

Beiser, M. (1985). A study of depression among traditional Africans, urban North Americans, and Southeast Asian refugees. In A. Kleinman & B. Good (Eds.), *Culture and depression* (p. 272). Berkeley: University of California Press.

Beiser, M., Benfari, R.C., Collomb, H., & Ravel, J. (1976). Measuring psychoneurotic behaviour in cross-cultural surveys. *Journal of Nervous and Mental Disease, 163,* 10–23.

Beiser, M., Cargo, M., & Woodbury, M. (1994). A comparison of psychiatric disorder in different cultures: Depressive typologies in South-East Asian refugees and resident Canadians. *International Journal of Methods in Psychiatric Research, 4,* 157–172.

Beiser, M. & Fleming, J.A.E. (1986). Measuring psychiatric disorder among Southeast Asian refugees. *Psychological Medicine, 16,* 627–640.

Beiser, M., Ravel, J., Collomb, H., & Egelhoff, C. (1972). Assessing psychiatric disorder among the Serer of Senegal. *Journal of Nervous and Mental Disease, 154,* 141–151.

Ben-Tovim, D.I. (1985). Therapy managing in Botswana. *Australian and New Zealand Journal of Psychiatry, 19,* 88–91.

Ben-Tovim, D.I. (1987). *Development psychiatry: Mental health and primary health care in Botswana.* London: Tavistock Publications.

Ben-Tovim, D.I. & Boyce, G.P. (1988). A comparison between patients admitted to psychiatric hospitals in Botswana and South Australia. *Acta Psychiatrica Scandinavica, 78,* 222–226.

Berger, R. (1995). Traditional healers. *British Medical Journal, 345,* 796.

Bertschy, G. & Ahyi, R.G. (1991). Obsessive–compulsive disorders in Benin: Five case reports. *Psychopathology, 24,* 398–401.

Binitie, A. (1981). Psychiatric disorders in a rural practice in the Bendel State of Nigeria. *Acta Psychiatrica Scandinavica, 64,* 273–280.

Binitie, A. (1991). The mentally ill in modern and traditional African societies. In S.O. Okpaku (Ed.), *Mental health in Africa and the Americas today* (p. 1). Nashville: Chrisolith Books.

Blue, I. & Harpham, T. (1994). The World Bank "World Development Report 1993": Investing in health. *British Journal of Psychiatry, 165,* 9–12.

Bourdillon, M. (1987). *The Shona peoples.* Gweru: Mambo Press.

Bourguignon, E. (1989). Competition and complementarity in the utilization of health resources in Africa. In K. Peltzer & P. Ebigbo (Eds.), *Clinical psychology in Africa* (p. 107). Enugu, Nigeria: Chuka Printing Company.

Bravo, M., Canino, G.J., Rubio-Stipec, M., & Woodbury-Farina, M. (1991). A cross-cultural adaptation of a psychiatric epidemiologic instrument: The Diagnostic Interview Schedule's adaptation in Puerto Rico. *Culture, Medicine and Psychiatry, 15,* 1–18.

Bridges, K. & Goldberg, D. (1985). Somatic presentations of DSM-III psychiatric disorders in primary care. *Journal of Psychosomatic Research, 29,* 563–569.

Bridges, K., Goldberg, D., Evans, B., & Sharpe, T. (1991). Determinants of somatization in primary care. *Psychological Medicine, 21,* 473–483.

Carothers, J. (1953). *The African mind in health and disease.* World Health Organisation Monograph 17. Geneva: WHO.

Cavender, A.P. (1991). Traditional medicine and an inclusive model of health seeking behaviour in Zimbabwe. Review. *Central African Journal of Medicine, 37,* 362–369.

Central Statistical Office (1995). *Zimbabwe National Census 1992*. Harare: Central Statistical Office.

Chandiwana, S.K. (1992). Development of health systems research and national HSR networking in Zimbabwe. *The Central African Journal of Medicine, 38*, 293–297.

Channabasavanna, S.M., Raguram, R., Weiss, M., Parvathavardhini, R., & Thriveni, M. (1993). Ethnography of psychiatric illness: A pilot study. *NIMHANS Journal, 11*, 1–10.

Chaturvedi, S. (1993). Neurosis across cultures. *International Review of Psychiatry, 5*, 179–191.

Chavunduka, G.L. (1978). *Traditional healers and the Shona patient*. Gwelo: Mambo Press.

Chavunduka, G.L. (1982). *Witches, witchcraft and the law in Zimbabwe*. ZINATHA Occasional Paper No. 1. Harare.

Chavunduka, G.L. (1986). ZINATHA: The organisation of traditional medicine in Zimbabwe. In M. Last & G.L. Chavunduka (Eds.), *The professionalisation of African medicine* (p. 29). Manchester: Manchester University Press.

Chavunduka, G.L. (1994). *Traditional medicine in modern Zimbabwe*. Harare: University of Zimbabwe Press,

Cheetham, R.W.S. & Cheetham, R.J (1976). Concepts of mental illness amongst the rural Xhosa people in South Africa. *Australian and New Zealand Journal of Psychiatry, 10*, 39–45.

Cheetham, R.W.S. & Griffiths, J.A. (1980). Changing patterns in psychiatry in Africa. *South African Medical Journal, 58*, 166–168.

Cheetham, R.W.S. & Griffiths, J.A. (1982). The traditional healer/diviner as psychotherapist. *South African Medical Journal, 62*, 957–958.

Cheetham, R.W.S. & Rzadkowolski, A. (1980). Crosscultural psychiatry and the concept of mental illness. *South African Medical Journal, 58*, 320–325.

Cheng, T.A. (1989). Symptomatology of minor psychiatric morbidity: A crosscultural comparison. *Psychological Medicine, 19*, 697–708.

Cheng, T.A. & Williams, P. (1986). The design and development of a screening questionnaire (CHQ) for use in community studies of mental disorders in Taiwan. *Psychological Medicine, 16*, 415–422.

Chikara, G. & Manley, M.R.S. (1991). Psychiatry in Zimbabwe. *Hospital and Community Psychiatry, 42*, 943–947.

City of Harare Health Department (1994). *Annual Report 1993*. Harare: City of Harare Health Department.

Compton, W.M., Helzer, J.E., Hwu, H.G., Yeh, E.K., McEvoy, L., Tipp, J.E., & Spitznagel, E.L. (1991). New methods in cross-cultural psychiatry: Psychiatric illness in Taiwan and the United States. *American Journal of Psychiatry, 148*, 1697–1704.

Corin, E. & Murphy, H.B.M. (1979). Psychiatric perspectives in Africa. Part 1: The Western viewpoint. *Transcultural Psychiatric Research Review, 16*, 147–178.

Dauskardt, R.P.A. (1990). Traditional medicine: Perpectives and policies in health care development. *Development Southern Africa, 7*, 351–358.

de Jong, J. (1987). *A descent into African psychiatry*. The Netherlands: Royal Tropical Institute.

de Jong, J., De Klein, G., & Ten Horn, S. (1986). A baseline study on mental disorders in Guinea-Bissau. *British Journal of Psychiatry, 148*, 27–32.

Dhadphale, M., Cooper, G., & Cartwright-Taylor, L. (1989). Prevalence and presentation of depressive illness in a primary health care setting in Kenya. *American Journal of Psychiatry, 146*, 659–661.

Dhadphale, M., Ellison, R.H., & Griffin, L. (1983). The frequency of psychiatric disorders among patients attending semi-urban and rural general out-patient clinics in Kenya. *British Journal of Psychiatry, 142,* 379–383.

Diop, B., Collignon, R., Gueye, M., & Harding, T.W. (1982). Diagnosis and symptoms of mental disorder in a rural area of Senegal. *African Journal of Medicine and Medical Science, 11,* 95–103.

Draguns, J. (1984). Assessing mental health and disorder across cultures. In P. Pedersen, N. Sartorius & A. Marsella (Eds.), *Mental health services: The cross-cultural context* (p. 31). London: Sage Publications.

Ebigbo, P.O. (1982). Development of a culture specific (Nigeria) screening scale of somatic complaints indicating psychiatric disturbance. *Culture, Medicine and Psychiatry, 6,* 29–43.

Ebigbo, P.O. (1986). The mind, the body, and society: An African perspective. *Advances: Institute for the Advancement of Health, 3,* 45–57.

Ebigbo, P.O., Janakiramaiah, N., & Kumaraswamy, N. (1989). Somatization in cross-cultural perspective. In K. Peltzer & P. Ebigbo (Eds.), *Clinical psychology in Africa* (p. 233). Enugu, Nigeria: Chuka Printing.

Edgerton, R.B. (1980). Traditional treatment for mental illness in Africa: A review. *Culture, Medicine and Psychiatry, 4,* 167–189.

Edwards, S.D., Grobbelaar, P.W., Makunga, N.V., Sibaya, P.T., Nene, L.M., Kunene, S.T., & Magwaza, A.S. (1983). Traditional Zulu theories of illness in psychiatric patients. *Journal of Social Psychology, 121,* 213–221.

Eisenbruch, M. (1990). Classification of natural and supernatural causes of mental distress. *Journal of Nervous and Mental Disease, 178,* 712–719.

Eisenbruch, M. (1991). From post-traumatic stress disorder to cultural bereavement: Diagnosis of Southeast Asian refugees. *Social Science and Medicine, 33,* 673–680.

Erinosho, O.A. & Ayonrinde, A. (1978). A comparative study of opinion and knowledge about mental illness in different societies. *Psychiatry, 41,* 403–410.

Essex, B. & Gosling, H. (1983). An algorithmic method for management of mental health problems in developing countries. *British Journal of Psychiatry, 143,* 451–459.

Fanuel, N. (1992). Knowledge, attitudes and practices of traditional healers in Gutu District. *Directory of Socio-Behavioural Research on HIV Infection and AIDS in Zimbabwe* (Abstract), 51–52.

Fernando, S. (1991). *Mental health, race and culture.* London: MIND and Macmillan.

Flaherty, J.A., Gaviria, F.M., Pathak, D., Mitchell, T., Wintrob, R., Richman, J.A., & Birz, S. (1988). Developing instruments for cross-cultural psychiatric research. *Journal of Nervous and Mental Disease, 176,* 257–263.

Fosu, G.B. (1981). Disease classification in rural Ghana: Framework and implications for health behaviour. *Social Science and Medicine, 15B,* 471–482.

Foulks, E.F., Persons, J.B., & Merkel, R.L. (1986). The effect of patients' beliefs about their illness on compliance with psychotherapy. *American Journal of Psychiatry, 143,* 340–344.

Freeman, M. (1991). An evaluation of mental health services in South Eastern Transvaal. In Centre for Health Policy (Ed.), *A Review of Health Services in Kangwane and the South Eastern Transvaal* (Vol. 10) (p. 28). Johannesburg: Department of Community Health, University of Witwatersrand.

Frye, B. & D'Avanzo, C. (1994). Themes in managing culturally defined illness in the Cambodian refugee family. *Journal of Community Health Nursing, 11,* 89–98.

Gelfand, M. (1964). Psychiatric disorders as recognized by the Shona. In A. Kiev (Ed.), *Magic, faith and healing* (p. 156). New York: Free Press.

Gelfand, M. (1967). Psychiatric disorders as recognized by the Shona. *Central African Journal of Medicine, 13,* 39–46.

Gelfand, M., Mavi, C.S., Drummond, R.B., & Ndemera, B. (1985). *The traditional medical practitioner in Zimbabwe*. Gweru: Mambo Press.

German, G.A. (1987). Mental health in Africa: 1. The extent of mental health problems in Africa today. *British Journal of Psychiatry, 151*, 435–439.

Giel, R. (1982). An epidemiological approach to the improvement of mental health services in developing countries. *Acta Psychiatrica Scandinavica, Suppl. 296, 65*, 56–63.

Giel, R. & Van Luijk, J.N. (1969). Psychiatric morbidity in a small Ethiopian town. *British Journal of Psychiatry, 115*, 149–162.

Gillis, L.S., Lewis, J.B., & Slabbert, M. (1968). Psychiatric disorder amongst the coloured people of the Cape Peninsula. *British Journal of Psychiatry, 114*, 1575–1587.

Goldberg, D. (1978). *Manual of the General Health Questionnaire*. Windsor: NFER.

Goldberg, D., Cooper, B., Eastwood, M., Kedward, H., & Shepherd, M. (1970). Standardized psychiatric interview for use in community surveys. *British Journal of Preventive and Social Medicine, 24*, 18–23.

Goldberg, D. & Huxley, P. (1992). *Common mental disorders: A biosocial model*. London: Tavistock/Routledge.

Goldberg, D. & Lecrubier, Y. (1995). Form and frequency of mental disorders across cultures. In T.B. Ustun & N. Sartorius (Eds.), *Mental illness in general health care: An international study* (p. 323). Chichester: Wiley.

Good, B.J., Good, M.D., & Moradi, R. (1985). The interpretation of Iranian depressive illness and dysphoric affect. In A. Kleinman & B. Good (Eds.), *Culture and depression* (p. 369). Berkeley: University of California Press.

Good, C.M. (1987). *Ethnomedical systems in Africa: Patterns of traditional medicine in rural and urban Kenya*. London: Guilford Press.

Gureje, O. & Obikoya, B. (1992). Somatization in primary care: Pattern and correlates in a clinic in Nigeria. *Acta Psychiatrica Scandinavica, 86*, 223–227.

Hall, A. & Williams, H. (1987). Hidden psychiatric morbidity: I. A study of prevalence in an outpatient population at Bindura Provincial Hospital. *Central African Journal of Medicine, 33*, 239–242.

Harding, T.W. (1975). Traditional healing methods for mental disorders. *WHO Chronicle, 31*, 436–440.

Harding, T.W., De Arango, M.V., Baltazar, J., Climent, C.E., Ibrahim, H.H.A., Ladrigo-Ignacio, L., Srinivasa Murthy, R., & Wig, N.N. (1980). Mental disorders in primary health care: A study of their frequency and diagnosis in four developing countries. *Psychological Medicine, 10*, 231–241.

Harpham, T. (1994). Urbanization and mental health in developing countries: A research role for social scientists, public health professionals and social psychiatrists. *Social Science and Medicine, 39*, 233–245.

Heggenhougen, K. & Draper, A. (1990). *Medical anthropology and primary health care*. EPC Publication No. 22, London School of Hygiene and Tropical Medicine, London.

Heggenhougen, K. & Sesia-Lewis, P. (1988). *Traditional medicine and primary health care*. EPC Publication No. 18, London School of Hygiene and Tropical Medicine, London.

Helman, C. (1981). Disease versus illness in general practice. *Journal of the Royal College of General Practitioners, 31*, 548–552.

Helman, C. (1985). Communication in primary care: The role of patient and practitioner explanatory models. *Social Science and Medicine, 20*, 923–931.

Helman, C. (1991). Limits of biomedical explanation. *Lancet, 337*, 1080–1082.

Hoff, W. & Nhlavana Maseko, D. (1986). Nurses and traditional healers join hands. *World Health Forum, 7*, 412–416.

Hollander, D. (1986). Zimbabwe: Mental health. *Lancet, July 26*, 212–213.

Hollifield, M., Katon, W., Spain, D., & Pule, L. (1990). Anxiety and depression in a village in Lesotho, Africa: A comparison with the United States. *British Journal of Psychiatry, 156,* 343–350.

Hunt, L., Jordan, B., & Irwin, S. (1989). Views of what's wrong: Diagnosis and patients' concept of illness. *Social Science and Medicine, 28,* 945–956.

Ihezue, U.H. (1989). The influence of sociocultural factors on symptoms of depression. In K. Peltzer & P. Ebigbo (Eds.), *Clinical psychology in Africa* (p. 217). Enugu, Nigeria: Chuka Printing.

Ilechukwu, S.T. (1988). Inter-relationships of beliefs about mental illness, psychiatric diagnoses and mental health care delivery among Africans. *The International Journal of Social Psychiatry, 34,* 200–206.

Jacob, K., Everitt, B., Patel, V., Welch, S., Araya, R., & Lewis, G.H. (1997). The comparison of latent variable models of non-psychotic morbidity in four culturally diverse populations. *Psychological Medicine* (in press).

Jahoda, G. (1961). Traditional healers and other institutions concerned with mental illness in Ghana. *International Journal of Social Psychiatry, 7,* 245–268.

Jegede, R.O. (1979). Depression in Africans revisited: A critical review of the literature. *African Journal of Medicine and Medical Science, 8,* 125–132.

Jegede, R.O., Ohaeri, J.U., Bamgboye, E.A., & Okunade, A.O. (1990). Psychiatric morbidity in a Nigerian general outpatient clinic. *West African Journal of Medicine, 9,* 177–186.

Jilek, W.G. (1993). Traditional medicine relevant to psychiatry. In N. Sartorius, G. de Girolamo, G. Andrews, G.A. German, & L. Eisenberg (Eds.), *Treatment of mental disorders: A review of effectiveness* (p. 341). Washington, DC: American Psychiatric Press.

Keegstra, H.J. (1986). Depressive disorders in Ethiopia. A standardized assessment using the SADD schedule. *Acta Psychiatrica Scandinavica, 73,* 658–664.

Kerson, D. & Jones, B. (1988). Tertiary care psychiatry in Zaire: DSM-III in the developing world. *International Journal of Social Psychiatry, 34,* 31–39.

Khan, M.E. & Manderson, L. (1992). Focus groups in tropical diseases research. *Health Policy and Planning, 7,* 56–66.

Kilonzo, G., Kaaya, S., Rweikiza, J., Kassam, M., & Moshi, G. (1994). Determination of appropriate clomipramine dosage among depressed African outpatients in Dar es Salaam, Tanzania. *Central African Journal of Medicine, 40,* 178–182.

Kinzie, J.D., Manson, S.M., Vinh, D.T., Tolan, N.T., Anh, B., & Pho, T.N. (1982). Development and validation of a Vietnamese-language depression rating scale. *American Journal of Psychiatry, 139,* 1276–1281.

Kirmayer, L.J. (1989). Cultural variations in the response to psychiatric disorders and emotional distress. *Social Science and Medicine, 29,* 327–339.

Kleinman, A. (1980). *Patients and healers in the context of culture.* Berkeley: University of California Press.

Kleinman, A. (1987). Anthropology and psychiatry: The role of culture in cross-cultural research on illness. *British Journal of Psychiatry, 151,* 447–454.

Kleinman, A. & Kleinman, J. (1985). Somatization: The interconnections in Chinese society among culture, depressive experiences, and the meanings of pain. In A. Kleinman & B. Good (Eds.), *Culture and depression* (p. 429). Berkeley: University of California Press.

Kortmann, F. (1987). Popular, traditional, and professional mental health care in Ethiopia. *Transcultural Psychiatric Research Review, 24,* 255–274.

Kortmann, F. & Ten Horn, S. (1988). Comprehension and motivation in responses to a psychiatric screening instrument: Validity of the SRQ in Ethiopia. *British Journal of Psychiatry, 153,* 95–101.

Krause, I-B. (1990). Cross-cultural psychiatric research: An anthropologist's view. *Psychiatric Bulletin, 14,* 143–146.

Kuyken, W., Orley, J., Hudelson, P., & Sartorius, N. (1994). Quality of life assessment across cultures. *International Journal of Mental Health, 23,* 5–28.

Lambo, T.A. (1969). Traditional African cultures and Western medicine. In F.N.L. Poynter (Ed.), *Medicine and culture* (p. 201). London: Wellcome Institute of the History of Medicine.

Lamont, A.M. (1988). Severe invalidism: The dominant feature of third-world psychiatry in southern Africa. *South African Medical Journal, 73,* 430–433.

Le Roux, A.G. (1973). Psychopathology in Bantu culture. *South African Medical Journal, 47,* 2077–2083.

Leff, J. (1977). The cross-cultural study of emotions. *Culture, Medicine and Psychiatry, 1,* 317–350.

Leff, J. (1990). The 'new cross-cultural psychiatry': A case of the baby and the bathwater. *British Journal of Psychiatry, 156,* 305–307.

Lefley, H. (1984). Delivering mental health services across cultures. In P. Pedersen, N. Sartorius, & A. Marsella (Eds.), *Mental health services: The cross-cultural context* (p. 135). London: Sage.

Leighton, A.H., Lambo, T.A., Hughes, C.C., Leighton, D.C., Murphy, J.M., & Macklin, D.B. (1963). *Psychiatric disorder among the Yoruba.* New York: Cornell University Press.

Lennock, J. (1994). *Paying for health: Poverty and structural adjustment in Zimbabwe.* Oxford: OXFAM Publication.

Lewis, G. (1991). Observer bias in the assessment of anxiety and depression. *Social Psychiatry and Psychiatric Epidemiology, 26,* 265–272.

Lewis, G. (1992). Dimensions of neurosis. *Psychological Medicine, 22,* 1011–1018.

Lewis, G., Pelosi, A., Araya, R., & Dunn, G. (1992). Measuring psychiatric disorder in the community: A standardized assessment for use by lay interviewers. *Psychological Medicine, 22,* 465–486.

Ley, P. (1988). *Communicating with patients.* London: Croom Helm.

Lin, T. (1983). Mental health in the third world. *Journal of Nervous and Mental Disease, 171,* 71–78.

Littlewood, R. (1990). From categories to contexts: A decade of the 'new cross-cultural psychiatry'. *British Journal of Psychiatry, 156,* 308–327.

Littlewood, R. (1991). From disease to illness and back again. *Lancet, 337,* 1013–1015.

Lloyd, K., Patel, V., Mann, A., Jacob, K., & St.Louis, L. (1996). A brief questionnaire to elicit health beliefs in common mental disorder (Abstract). *Winter meeting of the Royal College of Psychiatrists.*

Logie, D.E. & Woodroffe, J. (1993). Structural adjustment: The wrong prescription for Africa? *British Medical Journal, 307,* 41–43.

Lutz, C. (1985). Depression and the translation of emotional worlds. In A. Kleinman & B. Good (Eds.), *Culture and depression* (p. 63). Berkeley: University of California Press.

Majodina, M.Z. & Attah Johnson, F.Y. (1983). Standardized assessment of depressive disorders (SADD) in Ghana. *British Journal of Psychiatry, 143,* 442–446.

Makanjuola, R.O. (1987). "Ode Ori": A culture-bound disorder with prominent somatic features in Yoruba Nigerian patients. *Acta Psychiatrica Scandinavica, 75,* 231–236.

Makanjuola, R.O. & Jaiyeola, A.A. (1987). Yoruba traditional healers in psychiatry. II. Management of psychiatric disorders. *African Journal of Medicine and Medical Science, 16,* 61–73.

Makanjuola, J.D. & Olaifa, E.A. (1987). Masked depression in Nigerians treated at the Neuro-Psychiatric Hospital Aro, Abeokuta. *Acta Psychiatrica Scandinavica, 76,* 480–485.

Manson, S.M., Shore, J.H., & Bloom, J.D. (1985). The depressive experience in American Indian communities: A challenge for psychiatric theory and diagnosis. In A. Kleinman & B. Good (Eds.), *Culture and depression* (p. 331). Berkeley: University of California Press.

Mari, J., Sen, B., & Cheng, T.A. (1989). Case definition and case identification in cross-cultural perspective. In P. Williams, G. Wilkinson, & K. Rawnsley (Eds.), *The scope of epidemiological psychiatry* (p. 489). London: Routledge.

Mari, J. & Williams, P. (1985). A comparison of the validity of two psychiatric screening questionnaires (GHQ-12 and SRQ-20) in Brazil, using relative operating characteristic (ROC) analysis. *Psychological Medicine, 15*, 651–659.

Mari, J. & Williams, P. (1986). Misclassification by psychiatric screening questionnaires. *Journal of Chronic Disease, 39*, 371–378.

Marsella, A. & Westermeyer, J. (1993). Cultural aspects of treatment: Conceptual, methodological, and clinical issues and directions. In N. Sartorius, G. de Girolamo, G. Andrews, G.A. German, & L. Eisenberg (Eds.), *Treatment of Mental Disorders: a review of effectiveness* (p. 391). Washington: American Psychiatric Press.

Martyns-Yellowe, I. (1995). The development of a culture specific screening questionnaire NSRQ20 for use in psychiatric epidemiology: A preliminary report. *Culture, Medicine and Psychiatry, 19*, 113–123.

Morakinyo, O. (1985). Phobic states presenting as somatic complaints syndromes in Nigeria: Socio-cultural factors associated with diagnosis and psychotherapy. *Acta Psychiatrica Scandinavica, 71*, 356–365.

Morakinyo, O. (1989). Phobic states presenting as somatic complaints syndromes in Nigeria. In K. Peltzer & P. Ebigbo (Eds.), *Clinical Psychology in Africa* (p. 303). Enugu, Nigeria: Chuka Printing.

Mossop, R.T. & Stratford, G.A.C. (1986). Zimbabwe. In J. Fry & J.C. Hasler (Eds.), *Primary health care 2000* (p. 323). Edinburgh: Churchill Livingstone.

Mumford, D.B. (1993). Somatization: A transcultural perspective. *International Review of Psychiatry, 5*, 231–242.

Mumford, D.B., Bavington, J.T., Bhatnagar, K.S., Hussain, Y., Mirza, S., & Naraghi, M.M. (1991a). The Bradford Somatic Inventory: A multiethnic inventory of somatic symptoms reported by anxious and depressed patients in Britain and the Indo-Pakistan subcontinent. *British Journal of Psychiatry, 158*, 379–386.

Mumford, D.B., Tareen, I.A.K., Bajwa, M.A.Z., Bhatti, M.R., & Karim, R. (1991b). The translation and evaluation of an Urdu version of the Hospital Anxiety and Depression Scale. *Acta Psychiatrica Scandinavica, 83*, 81–85.

Murdock, G.P., Wilson, S.F., & Frederick, V. (1980). World distribution of theories of illness. *Transcultural Psychiatric Research Review, 17*, 37–64.

Murphy, H.B.M. (1977). Transcultural psychiatry should begin at home. *Psychological Medicine, 7*, 369–371.

Murphy, J. (1976). Psychiatric labeling in cross-cultural perspective. *Science, 191*, 1019–1028.

Mutambirwa, J. (1989). Health problems in rural communities, Zimbabwe. *Social Science and Medicine, 29*, 927–932.

Myambo, K. (1990). Social values and community development in rural Africa. *International Journal of Psychology, 25*, 767–777.

Mynors-Wallis, L., Gath, D., Lloyd-Thomas, A., & Tomlinson, D. (1995). Randomized controlled trial comparing problem solving with amitryptiline and placebo for major depression in primary care. *British Medical Journal, 310*, 441–445.

Nations, M., Camino, L., & Walker, F. (1988). Nerves: Folk idiom for anxiety and depression? *Social Science and Medicine, 26*, 1245–1259.

Ndetei, D.M. (1987). The association and implications of anxiety and depression in university medical and paramedical students in Kenya. *East African Medical Journal, 64*, 214–226.

Ndetei, D.M. & Muhangi, J. (1979). The prevalence and clinical pesentation of psychiatric illness in a rural setting in Kenya. *British Journal of Psychiatry, 135*, 269–272.

Neki, J.S., Joinet, B., Ndosi, N., Kilonzo, G., Hauli, J.G., & Duvinage, G. (1986). Witch-craft and psychotherapy. *British Journal of Psychiatry, 149*, 145–155.

Ngwenya, N. (1992). The role of the traditional health sector: An educational concern. *Allied health and health education: Multidisciplinary approaches* (p. 58). Ministry of Health, Kingdom of Swaziland and Kellogg Foundation, Piggs Peak, Swaziland.

Nhachi, C.F. & Kasilo, O.M. (1992). The pattern of poisoning in urban Zimbabwe. *Journal of Applied Toxicology, 12*, 435–438.

Nyamwaya, D. (1992). *African indigenous medicine.* Nairobi: African Medical and Research Foundation.

Nzewi, E. (1989). Cultural factors in the classification of psychopathology in Nigeria. In K. Peltzer & P. Ebigbo (Eds.), *Clinical psychology in Africa* (p. 208). Enugu, Nigeria: Chuka Printing.

Obeyesekere, G. (1985). Depression, Buddhism, and the work of culture in Sri Lanka. In A. Kleinman & B. Good (Eds.), *Culture and depression* (p. 134). Berkeley: University of California Press.

Obot, I. (1989). Public attitudes to and beliefs about psychosocial disorders. In K. Peltzer & P. Ebigbo (Eds.), *Clinical Psychology in Africa* (p. 103). Enugu, Nigeria: Chuka Printing.

Odejide, A.O. (1979). Cross-cultural psychiatry: A myth or reality. *Comprehensive Psychiatry, 20*, 103–109.

Odejide, A.O., Olatawura, M., Sanda, A., & Oyenye, A. (1977). Traditional healers and mental illness in the city of Ibadan. *African Journal of Psychiatry, 3*, 991–106.

Odejide, A.O., Oyewumi, L.K., & Ohaeri, J.U. (1989). Psychiatry in Africa: An overview. *American Journal of Psychiatry, 146*, 708–716.

Oduwole, O. & Ogunyemi, A.O. (1984). Psychiatric morbidity in a general medical clinic in Nigeria. *East African Medical Journal, 61*, 748–751.

Olatawura, M. (1982). Epidemiological psychiatry in Africa. *Acta Psychiatrica Scandinavica, Suppl. 296, 65*, 52–55.

Onyemelukwe, G., Ahmed, M.H., & Onyewotu, I. (1987). A survey of depressive symptomatology in Nigerians. *East African Medical Journal, 64*, 140–149.

Orley, J. & Wing, J.K. (1979). Psychiatric disorder in two African villages. *Archives of General Psychiatry, 36*, 513–520.

Ormel, J., Von Korff, M., Ustun, T., Pini, S., Korten, A., & Oldehinkel, T. (1994). Common mental disorders and disability across cultures. *Journal of the American Medical Association, 272*, 1741–1748.

Ormel, J., Von Korff, M., Van Den Brink, W., Katon, W., Brilman, E., & Oldehinkel, T. (1993). Depression, anxiety, and social disability show synchrony of change in primary care patients. *American Journal of Public Health, 83*, 385–390.

Otakpor, A.N. (1987). A prospective study of panic disorder in a Nigerian psychiatric outpatient population. *Acta Psychiatrica Scandinavica, 76*, 541–544.

Parry, C. (1996). A review of psychiatric epidemiology in Africa: Strategies for increasing validity when using instruments transculturally. *Transcultural Psychiatric Research Review, 33*, 173–188.

Patel, V. (1995a). Explanatory models of mental illness in sub-Saharan Africa. *Social Science and Medicine, 40*, 1291–1298.

Patel, V. (1995b). Spiritual distress: An indigenous concept of non-psychotic mental disorder in Harare. *Acta Psychiatrica Scandinavica, 92*, 103–107.

Patel, V. (1996). Recognizing common mental disorders in primary care in African countries: should "mental" be dropped? *Lancet, 347*, 742–744.

Patel, V., Gwanzura, F., Simunyu, E., Lewis, G., & Mann, A. (1997b). The Shona Symptom Questionnaire: The development of an indigenous measure of non-psychotic mental disorder in Harare. *Acta Psychiatrica Scandinavica, 95*, 469–475.

Patel, V., Gwanzura, F., Simunyu, E., Lloyd, K., & Mann, A. (1995d). The explanatory models and phenomenology of common mental disorder in Harare, Zimbabwe. *Psychological Medicine, 25*, 1191–1199.

Patel, V. & Mann, A. (1997). Etic and emic criteria for non-psychotic mental disorder: A study of the CISR and care provider assessment in Harare. *Social Psychiatry and Psychiatric Epidemiology, 32*, 84–89.

Patel, V., Musara, T., Maramba, P., & Butau, T. (1995a). Concepts of mental illness and medical pluralism in Harare. *Psychological Medicine, 25*, 485–493.

Patel, V., Mutambirwa, J., & Nhiwatiwa, S. (1995b). Stressed, depressed or bewitched: A perspective on mental illness, religion and culture. *Development in Practice, 5*, 216–224.

Patel, V., Simunyu, E., & Gwanzura, F. (1995c). Kufungisisa (thinking too much): A Shona idiom for non-psychotic mental illness. *Central African Journal of Medicine, 41*, 209–215.

Patel, V., Simunyu, E., & Gwanzura, F. (1997a). The pathways to primary mental health care in Harare, Zimbabwe. *Social Psychiatry and Psychiatric Epidemiology, 32*, 97–103.

Patel, V. & Todd, C.H. (1996). The validity of the Shona version of the Self-Report Questionnaire (SRQ) and the development of the SRQ8. *International Journal of Methods in Psychiatric Research, 6*, 153–160.

Patel, V., Todd, C., Winston, M., Gwanzura, F., Simunyu, E., Acuda, W., & Mann, A. (1997c). Common mental disorders in primary care in Harare, Zimbabwe: Associations and risk factors. *British Journal of Psychiatry, 171*, 60–64.

Patel, V., Todd, C., Winston, M., Gwanzura, F., Simunyu, E., Acuda, W., & Mann, A. (1997d). The outcome of common mental disorders in Harare. *British Journal of Psychiatry* (in press).

Patel, V. & Winston, M. (1994). The "universality" of mental disorder revisited: Assumptions, artefacts and new directions. *British Journal of Psychiatry, 165*, 437–440.

Paykel, E. & Priest, R. (1992). Recognition and management of depression in general practice: A consensus statement. *British Medical Journal, 305*, 1198–1202.

Peltzer, K. ((1988). The role of traditional and faith healers in primary mental health care: A Southern African perspective. *Curare, 11*, 207–210.

Peltzer, K. (1989). Spirit disorder in Malawi. In K. Peltzer & P. Ebigbo (Eds.), *Clinical Psychology in Africa* (p. 297). Enugu, Nigeria: Chuka Printing.

Pretorius, H. (1995). Mental disorders and disability across cultures: A view from South Africa. *Lancet, 345*, 534.

Reeler, A.P. (1986). Psychological disorders in Africa. Part 1: Issues of prevalence. *Central African Journal of Medicine, 32*, 298–302.

Reeler, A.P. (1992). Pathways to psychiatric care in Harare, Zimbabwe. *Central African Journal of Medicine, 38*, 1–7.

Reeler, A.P., Williams, H., & Todd, C.H. (1993). Psychopathology in primary care patients: A four year study in rural and urban settings in Zimbabwe. *The Central African Journal of Medicine, 39*, 1–7.

Roemer, M.I. (1991). Zimbabwe. In M.I. Roemer (Ed.), *National health systems of the world: The countries* (Vol. 1) (p. 540). Oxford: Oxford University Press.

Romme, M.A.J. (1987). Social psychiatry in Zimbabwe or the interplay of culture and psychosocial disorders. *International Journal of Social Psychiatry, 33*, 263–269.

Sartorius, N. (1986). Cross-cultural research on depression. *Psychopathology, 19, Suppl 2*, 6–11.

Sartorius, N. (1993). SCAN translation. In J. Wing, N. Sartorius, & T.B. Ustun (Eds.), *Diagnosis and clinical measurements in psychiatry: A reference manual for the SCAN system*. London: Cambridge University Press.

Sen, B. & Mari, J. (1986). Psychiatric research instruments in the transcultural setting: Experiences in India and Brazil. *Social Science and Medicine, 23*, 277–281.

Sharp, L. (1994). Exorcists, psychiatrists, and the problems of possession in Northwest Madagascar. *Social Science and Medicine, 38*, 525–542.

Sims, A. (1994). "Psyche": Spirit as well as mind? *British Journal of Psychiatry, 165*, 441–446.

Srinivasan, T.N. & Suresh, T.R. (1990). Non-specific symptoms and screening of non-psychotic morbidity in primary care. *Indian Journal of Psychiatry, 32*, 77–82.

Staugard, F. (1985). *Traditional medicine in Botswana: Traditional healers.* Gaborone: Ipelegeng.

Stock, R. (1995). *Africa south of the Sahara: A geographical interpretation.* New York: Guilford.

Stott, R., Mombe, C.S., Meijer, F., Nyadzema, N., & Zhangu, C.S. (1988). Is cooperation between traditional and Western healers possible? A pilot study from Zimbabwe. *Complementary Medical Research, 3*, 15–22.

Suresh, T.R., Suresh Kumar, M., Bashyam, V.S., & Srinivasan, T.N. (1993). The nonspecific symptom screening method: A replication study. *Indian Journal of Psychiatry, 35*, 151–153.

Swartz, L. (1986). Transcultural psychiatry in South Africa (Part 1). *Transcultural Psychiatric Research Review, 23*, 273–303.

Swartz, L. (1987). Transcultural psychiatry in South Africa (Part 2). *Transcultural Psychiatric Research Review, 24*, 5–30.

Swartz, L., Ben-Arie, O., & Teggin, A. (1985). Subcultural delusions and hallucinations: comments on the present state examination in a multi-cultural context. *British Journal of Psychiatry, 146*, 391–394.

Tansella, M., de Girolamo, G., & Sartorius, N. (1992). *Annotated bibliography of psychiatric epidemiology.* London: Gaskell.

Tyrer, P. (1996). Comorbidity or cosanguinity. *British Journal of Psychiatry, 168*, 669–671.

Ugorji, R.U. & Ofem, O.U.E. (1976). The concept of mental illness among the Yakkur of Nigeria. *African Journal of Psychiatry, 2*, 295–298.

Ustun, T., Goldberg, D., Cooper, J., Simon, G., & Sartorius, N. (1995b). New classification for mental disorders with management guidelines for use in primary care: ICD-10 PHC chapter five. *British Journal of General Practice, 45*, 211–215.

Ustun, T. & Sartorius, N. (1995). The background and rationale of the WHO collaborative study on "psychological problems in general health care". In T.B. Ustun & N. Sartorius (Eds.), *Mental illness in general health care: An international study* (p. 1). Chichester: Wiley.

Ustun, T., Simon, G., & Sartorius, N. (1995a). Discussion. In T.B. Ustun & N. Sartorius (Eds.), *Mental illness in general health care: An international perspective* (p. 361). Chichester: Wiley.

Varkevisser, C.M., Pathmanathan, I., & Brownlee, A. (1991). *Designing and conducting health systems research projects:* Vol. 2, Part 2 (data analysis and report writing). Ottawa & Geneva: IDRC & WHO.

Velimirovic, B. (1992). Is integration of traditional and Western medicine really possible? In J. Coreil & J.D. Mull (Eds.), *Anthropology and primary health care* (p. 51). Boulder: Westview.

Venkoba Rao, A. (1994). Depressive disorder. *Social Science and Medicine, 38*, v–viii.

Von Korff, M., Ustun, T., Ormel, J., Kaplan, I., & Simon, G. (1996). Self-report disability in an international primary care study of psychological illness. *Journal of Clinical Epidemiology, 49*, 297–303.

Wessels, W.H. (1985). The traditional healer and psychiatry. *Australian and New Zealand Journal of Psychiatry, 19*, 283–286.

Westermeyer, J. (1985). Psychiatric diagnosis across cultural boundaries. *American Journal of Psychiatry, 142,* 798–805.

Westermeyer, J. (1989). Psychiatric epidemiology across cultures: Current issues and trends. *Transcultural Psychiatric Research Review, 26,* 5–25.

Williams, P., Tarnopolsky, A., & Hand, D. (1980). Case definition and case identification: Review and assessment. *Psychological Medicine, 10,* 101–114.

Wing, J.K., Cooper, J.E., & Sartorius, N. (1974). *The measurement and classification of psychiatric symptoms.* London: Cambridge University Press.

Winston, M. & Patel, V. (1995). Use of traditional and orthodox medicine in urban Zimbabwe. *International Journal of Epidemiology, 24,* 1006–1012.

Winston, M., Patel, V., Musonza, T., & Nyathi, Z. (1995). A community survey of traditional medical practitioners in Harare. *Central African Journal of Medicine, 41,* 278–283.

World Bank, (1993). *World development report.* Washington, DC: Oxford University Press.

World Health Organisation (1992). *The ICD-10 classification of mental and behavioural disorders.* Geneva: World Health Organisation.

World Health Organisation (1995). *The world health report 1995: Bridging the gaps.* Geneva: World Health Organisation.

Appendix 1

ITEM SOURCE OF THE PRELIMINARY SHONA SYMPTOM QUESTIONNAIRE

Items from preliminary SSQ only

Dizziness
Blackouts
Leg ache
Difficulty walking
Backache
Worries about life's problems
Worries about health
Thinking too much
Forgetfulness
Lack of concentration
Irritability
Feeling confused or as if losing one's mind
Feeling as if one's behaviour had changed
Feeling that one's blood pressure was high
Palpitations
Feeling suffocated or having difficulty in breathing
Chest/heartache
Other heart/chest sensations such as pricking and heaviness
Sharp pains in the sides
Feeling heat or cold sensations in the body
Nightmares or bad dreams
Loss of weight
Lacking in energy
Mabayo (a pricking side sensation)
Nausea and vomiting
Perceptual disturbances
Abdominal discomfort after meals
Sensations of things moving in the body
Abdominal pain
Pain in the navel region
Feeling as if veins are being pulled

Feelings of hopelessness
Excessive sweating
Shaking or trembling
Not feeling like speaking or being spoken to
Being easily startled by trivial things

Items in common with the preliminary SSQ and SRQ

Feeling panicky or getting startled
Difficulty sleeping or falling asleep
Tearfulness
Feeling unhappy or sad
Headaches
Loss of appetite
Tiredness
Suicidal ideas
Loss of interest

Items from the SRQ alone

Difficulty enjoying daily activities
Being unable to play a useful role in life
Feelings of worthlessness
Daily work suffering
Difficulty making decisions
Trouble thinking clearly
Feeling tense, nervous, or worried
Uncomfortable feelings in stomach
Poor digestion
Hands shaking
Easily tired

Items on positive mental health

Feeling happy with life
Seeing the future with hope and optimism
Clear thinking
Feeling contented

Appendix 2

ITEMS OF THE PRELIMINARY SSQ SELECTED FOR FURTHER ANALYSIS

Item	Source	Item	Source
Tearfulness	Comb.	Daily work suffering	SRQ
Poor sleep	Comb.	Nervous, tense, or worried	SRQ
Difficulty enjoying daily activities	SRQ	Perceptual symptoms, viz. hallucinations	pSSQ
Loss of interest in daily activities	Comb.	Lacking in energy	pSSQ
Don't feel like speaking to others	pSSQ	Irritability	pSSQ
Sadness	Comb.	Dizziness	pSSQ
Tiredness	Comb.	Disturbing dreams	pSSQ
Feeling hopeless	pSSQ	Loss of appetite	Comb.
Worthlessness	SRQ	Being easily startled	pSSQ
Difficulty making decisions	SRQ	Lack of concentration	pSSQ
Unable to play a useful part in life	SRQ	Stomach ache	pSSQ
Thinking too much	pSSQ	Difficulty breathing	pSSQ
Suicidal ideas	Comb.	Loss of weight	pSSQ
Feeling as if one had high blood pressure	pSSQ	Worrying about life's problems	pSSQ
Feeling as if one is going mad	pSSQ	*Mabayo* (pricking side sensation)	pSSQ
Palpitations	pSSQ	Leg ache	pSSQ

Key: SRQ = items derived from SRQ; pSSQ = items derived from preliminary SSQ; Comb. = items common to both sources.

Appendix 3

PATIENT VARIABLES ELICITED TO STUDY ASSOCIATIONS WITH COMMON MENTAL DISORDERS

Clinical variables and explanatory models
Reasons for consultation
Duration of illness
Number of presenting complaints
Causal model
Belief that witchcraft had caused illness
Belief that *kufungisisa* (thinking too much) had caused illness
Belief in somatic origin of illness
History of emotional problems/stress in previous year
Alcohol use

Sociodemographic variables
Sex
Age
Years of formal education
Educational qualifications
Occupation
Whether mother is dead
Whether father is dead
Marital status
Number of children
Whether subject has a rural home
Religion

Economic variables
Accommodation (owned/rented)
Crowding
Ownership of radio
Ownership of TV
Whether on social welfare
Whether on medical aid
Whether unable to buy food in the past month due to lack of money
Cash savings
Whether in debt and reasons for debt
Degree of stressfulness of debt

Life events in past 12 months
Marriage
Divorce/Separation
Pregnancy
Abortion
Infertility
Trouble with in-laws
Child leaving home
Husband takes a new wife (for women)
Retirement
Loss of job
Change of job
Spouse begins work
Spouse stops work
Sickness in family
Personal injury
Death of spouse
Death of child
Death of parent
Death of relative
Death of friend

Disability/impact of illness
Impact on daily life (open question)
Brief Disability Questionnaire score
Days off sick (from daily activities) in previous month
Days bedridden in previous month
Overall quality of life

Pathways to care
First care provider consulted
Consultations with 6 care provider types PHC, GP, Hospital, *n'anga*, *profita*, church priest) in previous 12 months
Number of consultations with these 6 care provider types in previous month

Author index

Subject index